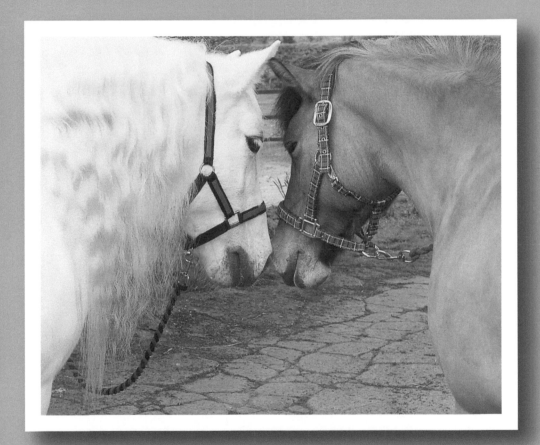

Horse
Senses

Susan McBane
Co-Founder, Equine Behaviour Forum
Co-Editor of Equine Behaviour (with Dr Francis Burton)

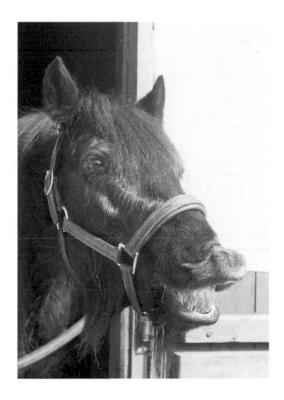

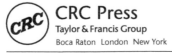

CRC Press
Taylor & Francis Group
Boca Raton London New York

CRC Press is an imprint of the
Taylor & Francis Group, an **informa** business

DEDICATION

To Pauline and Waverhead Rose (whose photo appears on the title page),
with many thanks for all the challenging rides.
' ... after all, she's only a Fell Pony!'

Front cover photo by David Watson of HORSEPIX of Megan, a Welsh Section D mare
owned by Caroline Lacey–Freeman

CRC Press
Taylor & Francis Group
6000 Broken Sound Parkway NW, Suite 300
Boca Raton, FL 33487-2742

First issued in paperback 2019

© 2012 by Taylor & Francis Group, LLC
CRC Press is an imprint of Taylor & Francis Group, an Informa business

No claim to original U.S. Government works

ISBN: 978-1-84076-080-4 (hbk)
ISBN: 978-0-376-38177-6 (pbk)

Visit the Taylor & Francis Web site at
http://www.taylorandfrancis.com

and the CRC Press Web site at
http://www.crcpress.com

A CIP catalogue record for this book is available from the British Library.

CONTENTS

DISCLAIMER

The content of this book is provided for interest and information. The publisher and author cannot be held responsible in any way for the results of applying the techniques or using the information contained herein. The information is accurate to the best of their knowledge and belief. This book is not intended as a substitute for or to replace professional help. Its purpose is to help readers to understand and help their horses, and to promote their welfare and health. Horses are unpredictable animals and associating with them is potentially dangerous. Readers should take appropriate safety precautions to safeguard themselves, their horses, other people and animals, and property in addition to taking out their own insurance.

ACKNOWLEDGEMENTS

I wish to thank Dr Francis Burton for the great amount of work he has put into helping me with this book. His generous and conscientious attitude has been very much appreciated and, combined with his knowledge and skills, has given this book an accuracy and authority that it could not otherwise have had. If there are any remaining errors or inadequacies, they are mine and not his.

My thanks also go to my copy editor, Peter Beynon, who is a veterinary surgeon. This is the first time I have had my work copyedited by a vet and his technical knowledge of the subject has been a big help and reassurance to me, along with his light touch and tact.

My good friend Pauline Finch deserves my sincere appreciation for executing most of the line drawings in this book. She coped admirably not only with the task in hand, but also with my tendency to ask for drawings at very short notice, which she never failed to produce. She also generously made available her piebald, Sky, for some photographs. Their trainer, Jo Birkbeck, BHSII, also spent a good deal of time staging photographs and persuading Sky to come up with the goods, as did Vicky Gardner, who helps to look after him. Pauline's Fell Pony, Rose, to whom this book is dedicated and who appears on the title page, is my special friend and teacher, and she, too, had a hoof in several of the photographs, as did her companion, Shetland Pony Pip Finch.

Liz Whitehead and her handsome horse, Drummer, also spent a morning posing for photographs for which I was most grateful, and my sincere thanks also go to Betty Paul and her human and equine family and friends, who appear in several of the pictures.

Finally, my appreciation and thanks go to the team at Manson Publishing for their professionalism and expert assistance in bringing this book to fruition.

PREFACE

For thousands of years people have associated with horses, initially for solely practical purposes such as food and the use of their body parts and products (e.g. blood and milk), and later for transport and also as companions and friends. This is quite strange for two main reasons: firstly because horses are prey animals and humans are historically predators, and secondly because the horse does not perceive the world as we do. In fact, in several ways horses perceive it quite differently, and yet we have had the closest of relationships over the generations.

I imagine that many of the veterinary students who will read this book will never actually ride or drive a horse. I have always thought that not being able to ride and acquire that extra level of experience of such a large, working animal must create a disadvantage when it comes to treating his disorders, but on the other hand, perhaps non-riders have more sense than those of us who do ride! Others who read this book, such as equine science students and those who are planning a professional career with horses, will also be riders. In either case, I hope this survey and introduction to equine senses will help everyone to understand horses more and, in particular, understand why they behave in the ways they do, ways that very often confuse even the most experienced of horsemen and women.

We are very prone to dismissing horses' behaviour and our lack of comprehension of it with such phrases as 'It's just the way they are. We'll never really understand them.' This may be true, but surely we must try to do so as best we can, not only for our own enjoyment, knowledge and safety, but also for the horses' sakes. More and more, as scientific research goes on in the fields of equine behaviour, anatomy and physiology, we are coming to realise more clearly how horses work, and that is often very different from how we have traditionally believed them to function and to think. Many people still treat and train horses like human children, which is often not only highly inappropriate, but also potentially dangerous and abusive.

Maybe I should not say it in a book of this nature, but I do not think science has all the answers, although lay horse people do not, either. The best way forward is surely for us all to work together, for none of us to think that we know it all, and for our joint cooperation to result in greatly improved methods of working, caring for and managing horses from their point of view. Over the years, horses seem to have learned far better how to work with us than we have learned how to work with them. This is quite an indictment against humankind when one considers how long we have used and associated with horses and how many opportunities we have missed along the way.

By better appreciating life from the horse's viewpoint through understanding how his senses work and how he experiences our mutual world, I really hope we will realise what an exceptionally giving and, in his own way, smart animal we are associating with.

Susan McBane

INTRODUCTION

This book aims to bridge the gap between scientific textbooks and books for the general equestrian reader. I hope this will mean that it will be of use to horse enthusiasts with little or no scientific knowledge, to first year equine science and veterinary students, to those studying for professional equestrian examinations, equine studies degrees and other courses, and to committed owners wanting to relate science to practice. I have chosen the subject of the horse's senses because so little seems to have been written about them in the general equestrian literature. I have tried to present information as reasonably up to date as I can according to the state of both scientific and practical knowledge at the time of writing, bearing in mind that research is an ongoing process that constantly adds to our knowledge, understanding and viewpoint of horses.

Horses are extremely sensitive, perceptive animals, classic examples of grazing, running prey animals with an intelligence developed in and geared towards their natural environment, but with the added bonus of tremendous adaptability. They are very strong in comparison with other species of similar body size, they are fast and they are often easily trained depending not only on their propensities as a species but also on individual inclinations tempered by past experience and current management and state of mind.

Although initially used by man for food and ancillary purposes – every part of the body being useful for something – their combined qualities of strength, size, speed, sociability, trainability and adaptability and, in many cases, beauty were fairly quickly realised and valued, being found together in no other animal (1). Horses are often inquisitive and many of them seem to actually want to be with us and to learn what we want to teach them once they know and trust us.

The senses of horses are highly developed, particularly those of hearing and smell. Most animal species seem to have more effective senses than humans, who seem to be particularly deficient in the ability to smell and hear as sharply as others.

Not all the horse's qualities work in our favour, though. As a species, they are suspicious and cautious, features that have contributed greatly towards their survival as prey animals for millions of years. They can be highly strung, often nervous and also highly reactive, depending not always on breed but often on individuality. They pay great attention to their environment and are particularly alert to even small changes in it – a tree blown down, a house painted a different colour, sheep in a field where they are not normally, a vehicle or people and animals moving in the far distance, roadworks or a newly ploughed field. Sometimes they react significantly to these changes; sometimes they appear to merely note them.

As horses live naturally in a wide, open world, their mind-set is not so 'close to home' as ours. They live mentally in a more far-reaching environment than we do; they look a much greater distance ahead and around than we do; and they use their vision, which in particular is quite different from ours, and hearing to assess their

1 Although initially people had to deal with horses purely for practical reasons such as transport, haulage and food, it cannot have been long before affectionate relationships developed. Horses are herd animals with strong bonds with their family and other herd members, but they are just as happy to associate with humans in most cases, provided they are treated well.

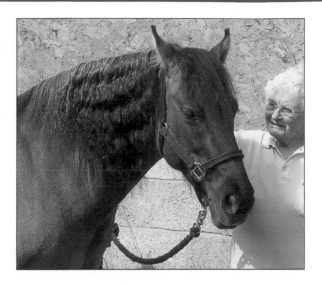

surroundings for apparently miles around. These evolutionary traits mean that horses can take in many of the features of their locale that are not recognized by humans. Being naturally wary, they may easily react to features, movements, sounds and even smells of which we are not even aware. Many a horse has been forcefully reprimanded by its rider or driver for being stubborn, flighty or stupid, when he was simply acting on information coming in from his superior senses, which warned him that he could be in danger.

Throughout this book I have concentrated on trying to perceive and convey the world as the horse seems to perceive it – something, of course, that it is impossible to do perfectly accurately because we can never get inside a horse's skin, never mind his head, and live as he does. However, from what we know to date (and there is a very great deal we still do not know) about a horse's senses, it is quite possible to hazard a reasonable guess at how they affect his behaviour and his viewpoint and experience of this world and this life we both share. This enables us to give him much more appropriate treatment in relation to his management and work, treatment that accords with the kind of animal he is.

COMPLEMENTARY THERAPIES

Some people call these therapies 'alternative' therapies, but I see them as absolutely complementary to veterinary practices and treatments and also, often, to each other. Complementary therapies can, of course, be used alone and so can what we currently regard as orthodox medicine, but my experience is that the two together often produce a synergistic effect.

Some readers of this book may be students of veterinary medicine and equine science and, as such, will be receiving conventional, 'hard science' training. They will be quite right, bearing that in mind, to query whether or not complementary therapies actually work. Increasingly, there is scientific evidence acceptable to the scientific community that some therapies do work; for example, herbalism and also acupuncture (and, by logical extrapolation, its related therapies of acupressure and shiatsu). A human generation ago, physiotherapy and osteopathy were regarded as 'quackery' and some doctors used to refer their patients privately 'under the table', as it were. Both therapies are now mainstream in many countries, and doctors give referrals to acupuncturists, homoeopaths and other therapists; this represents a real sea change in outlook.

In some countries a referral from a veterinary surgeon is needed before any other therapist is allowed to treat an animal. Also, in some countries, including the UK, only a veterinary surgeon is permitted, by law, to diagnose an animal's condition. Even if this is not the case, I feel that consulting your veterinary surgeon first on any aspect of your horse's health care is the best course of action, not least because of the rigorous all-round training vets receive in anatomy and physiology. As a trained equine shiatsu practitioner myself, I have never yet come across a veterinary surgeon who either belittled my therapy or would not allow me to treat a horse. Some vets are themselves trained and qualified in specific complementary therapies, notably homoeopathy, and a few are qualified in medical herbalism and other modalities. The world is changing, and a more open-minded attitude is much more evident in both human and animal medicine, and is expected by many patients and clients.

In Part 3 of this book (Management and Work), I have given some details of a complementary therapy that seems particularly appropriate for the sense under discussion. I hope this will encourage readers to look further into the whole field of complementary therapies in relation to management, health maintenance and healing.

EQUINE BEHAVIOUR

Everything a horse does comprises some kind of behaviour. It always amazes me that there are so many professional and amateur horse people who say that they are not particularly interested in equine behaviour as such. Everything we ask a horse to do is a request for a particular type of behaviour, from moving over in the stable or standing still for attention to hacking out safely, winning races or jumping formidable fences; therefore, everyone, whether they admit or realise it or not, is interested in equine behaviour.

Formal, traditional teaching organisations have only quite recently started to feature equine psychology and behaviour more in their syllabuses; however, the coverage still seems to be very sparse compared with other aspects of dealing with horses such as riding and general management. Despite this, people are very ready to complain when horses 'misbehave' or do not act as their human connections would wish. It is a sobering experience when you come to realise that most horses' behaviour problems are caused by the inappropriate management methods and training techniques inflicted on them by us humans.

A lot of the difficulty, I believe, is because it is still not generally or fully appreciated how differently from us a horse perceives the world. There is still a great deal we do not know regarding both the horse's senses and his behaviour. The latter is very often the result of his perception and assessment of something in his surroundings, something we may even be completely unaware of such as a high-pitched sound, ground vibrations, an interesting smell or something suspicious within the horse's field of vision but outside ours. His view of a fence, for instance, may be different from ours in both form and colour, so he may refuse a perfectly simple looking fence and is unable to tell us why (2).

There are many excellent books on equine behaviour itself (see Further Reading). This book concentrates on trying to describe the horse's senses, mainly in practical terms, and details how the horse's senses can be taken account of during management and training/working techniques, making for better understanding and, it is hoped, removing the confusion and frustration often currently experienced by both parties.

Horses meet us well over halfway in our lives together. There is so much more that we could do to repay their generosity and trust.

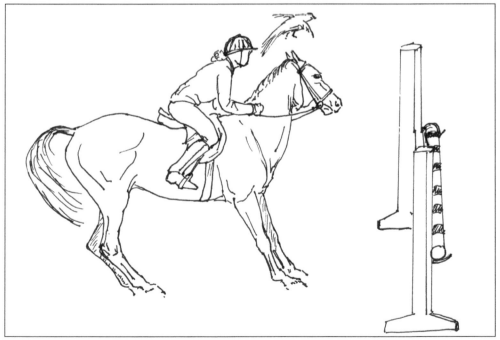

2 A horse may refuse an easy looking fence because his vision gives him a different view of it from our own. Something on the periphery of his field of vision, on the other side of the fence or even towards the rear extreme of his field of vision may discourage him from jumping.

THE EQUINE BEHAVIOUR FORUM

The Equine Behaviour Forum (EBF) was founded (as The Equine Behaviour Study Circle) in 1978 by the late Dr Moyra Williams (a clinical psychologist and renowned horsewoman and performance horse breeder) and the author of this book. It is an international, British-based forum, run on a voluntary and non-profit basis, for the exchange of information and opinions on equine behaviour and, as such, is not a formal teaching organisation. Its current Chairman and Scientific Editor is Dr Francis Burton of The University of Glasgow.

Written and illustrated almost entirely by its members, its quarterly journal, *Equine Behaviour*, is popular with scientists and lay readers, professional horse people and amateurs alike. It publishes articles, opinions, letters, book reviews, conference reports and similar features. The EBF presents a Scientific Symposium most years. More information can be obtained by visiting the EBF's website:

www.gla.ac.uk/external/EBF/

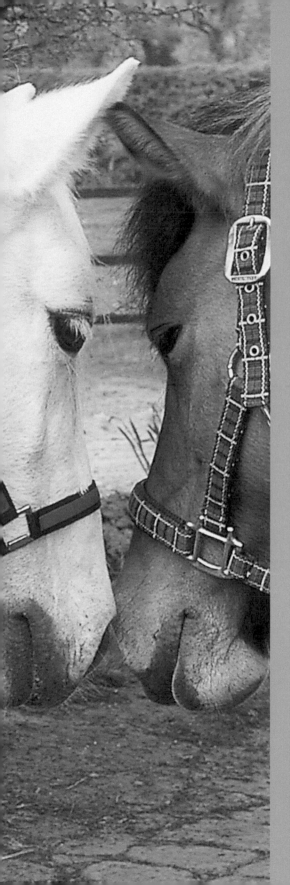

Part 1
General Anatomy and Physiology

The main control systems of the body are the nervous system and the endocrine/hormonal system. These two systems often work closely together in many different functions, ranging from the lightning reactions needed in cases of urgent self-preservation in the presence of danger to processes that sustain life in general such as digestion, the beating of the heart, breeding and many others.

Chapter 1:
The Nervous System

Chapter 2:
The Endocrine/Hormonal System

Chapter 1
THE NERVOUS SYSTEM

The nervous system is a complex and highly organised system of electrically active neurones or nerve cells that send and receive signals as electrical impulses. Stimuli from the environment and from the body itself are received and coordinated via sensory receptors, and commands are conveyed to glands (see The Endocrine/Hormonal System) and muscles so that the horse can sense and respond, often in a split second, to internal and external stimuli from light reflections and sound waves, to a rider's aids, to a potential predator approaching or to a kick from another horse.

The nervous system is divided into two parts: the central nervous system (CNS) comprising the brain and the spinal cord, and the peripheral nervous system (PNS) comprising the nerves and ganglia (masses of nerve cell bodies) branching from the CNS around the body.

THE CENTRAL NERVOUS SYSTEM

The brain, housed inside the cranial cavity of the skull, consists of soft, pinky-grey tissue, which is the main mass of ganglia in the body. The spinal cord runs from the brain down inside the backbone, which is formed by individual bones or vertebrae linked by pads of cartilage, the protein-rich protective pads found in many joints. Messages can be received and sent by both the brain and the spinal cord (**3a, b**).

THE PERIPHERAL NERVOUS SYSTEM

Branching out from the spinal cord through grooves between the vertebrae are many nerves. These are string-like structures consisting of a collection of nerve fibres or cells that carry messages or impulses to and fro all around the body, according to the purpose of the nerve. There are sensory and motor nerves, and also nerves known as mixed nerves because they can transmit messages both to and from the CNS.

The sensory function of the PNS is carried out by two types of nerve fibres, which sense conditions both inside and outside the body.

The motor nerves have a voluntary function that enables the horse to perform actions as, and if, he wishes. There is also an involuntary function, which the horse cannot control; this governs such matters as digestion, reproduction and heart function. Sometimes, the horse can take some control over this involuntary function, notably in the occasional control of breathing (such as sniffing to detect a smell) and mares can hold back on foaling to some extent until they judge the environment is safe. Generally, though, the involuntary function of the PNS is beyond the horse's control.

The peripheral nervous system is divided by function into the somatic nervous system and the autonomic nervous system.

The Somatic Nervous System

The somatic nervous system is responsible mainly for actions that are voluntary or under the control of the horse's will and that involve the contraction of skeletal muscles. The horse decides whether or not to wander over to a different patch of grass, to scratch his ear, comply with his rider's wishes or kick the vet.

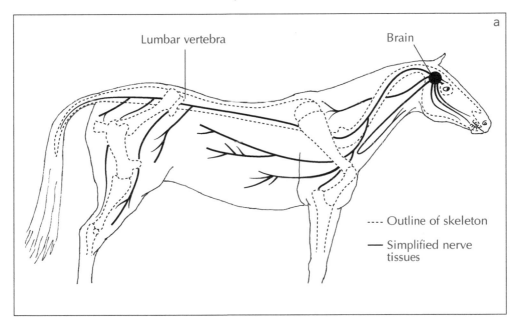

a

Lumbar vertebra

Brain

---- Outline of skeleton

— Simplified nerve tissues

3a, b (3a) Diagram showing how nerves branch out around the body from the spinal cord, which itself runs from the brain. (3b) Diagram of a lumbar vertebra showing how the spinal cord runs through the vertebrae along the spine, from the brain to approximately halfway down the dock.

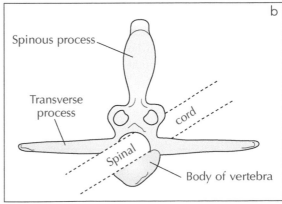

b

Spinous process

Transverse process

Spinal cord

Body of vertebra

The system has three main roles:

- **A sensory role.** The somatic nervous system detects/receives stimuli, via the horse's senses, from outside or inside the body. Examples of such stimuli include weather conditions, the presence of something suspicious or viewed as dangerous, the scent of a strange horse or one known to be unfriendly or a predator, a feeling of hunger or thirst, or an aid from the rider. The system then sends a message in the form of either a hormone (chemical messenger) or an electrical impulse along sensory (afferent) nerves to the brain and/or spinal cord, informing them of the type of stimulus it has received.
- **A directing role.** The CNS assesses the impulses or messages received and sends instructions to the relevant part or parts of the body about what to do in response, if anything.
- **A response or action role.** The instructions from the CNS are carried by electrical impulses down motor (efferent) nerves to the part or parts of the body concerned, telling them how to act in response to the stimuli.

The Autonomic Nervous System

The involuntary function of the PNS is itself split into two subdivisions, the parasympathetic nervous system and the sympathetic nervous system, together called the autonomic nervous system.

The **parasympathetic nervous system** has an energy conservation role and is therefore concerned with securing the body's resources.

The **sympathetic nervous system** has opposing functions to the parasympathetic nervous system, and is geared towards using up energy and protecting the horse. It is involved in the 'flight or fight' response when danger threatens, or appears to the horse to do so; therefore, in an animal like the horse, the sympathetic nervous system is in frequent use. It causes the horse to stop eating and drinking, to become alert and assess his surroundings and the behaviour of his herd mates and other birds and animals, and to check on the presence of any threat. The sympathetic nervous system is also involved in defence, whether against a rough rider or handler, an anti-social herd member or a predator. It speeds up the heart rate and respiratory rate and reduces gut movements, dilating blood vessels in the muscles as blood is redirected to them to fuel action. It also dilates the air passages for the inspiration of oxygen and expiration of carbon dioxide. Anything that involves the use of energy, from flicking the tail at a fly to jumping round a cross-country course, is a concern of the sympathetic system. Although the sympathetic nervous system is not necessary for life as such, it is an important modifier.

SUMMARY

The above is the received wisdom concerning the very basic functioning of the nervous system. However, Dr Tristan D.M. Roberts, former Reader in Physiology at The University of Glasgow, has made a personal study of nerve impulses and sensory messages, which gives a rather different view of the process. His book *Recollections of a Frustrated Scientist* (Roberts, 2006), gives considerable detail about his findings and opinions. As far as perception of nervous messages goes, Dr Roberts believes that because the electrical impulses travelling along the sensory nerves are the same, there is no way that the CNS can perceive what the messages mean to convey, therefore perception itself must be happening in some other way. For those interested in these topics, I recommend his book, which manages to be amusing, entertaining, fascinating, instructional and thought provoking all at the same time.

(More information on the structure and function of nerves and of reflexes is given in Part 3: Management and Work, The Sense of Touch.)

Chapter 2
THE ENDOCRINE/
HORMONAL SYSTEM

The endocrine system is responsible for the production, release and control of hormones within the body. Hormones are very underrated substances. They can be described simply as regulatory chemical transmitter substances or messengers aimed ultimately at promoting the survival of both the species in general and the individual in particular. The yearly cycle of hormones rising and falling control at what seasons of the year horses feel like mating, and the roughly three-week cycle of the mare (a wheel within a wheel) determines the progression of her oestrus cycles. Hormones are responsible for many functions of the horse's body and are usually not considered in this context by owners. The number of hormones is still not known, and each has a unique chemical formula and purpose.

The endocrine system works closely with the nervous system. Although it is the latter that initially, for instance, sets the horse in motion when he is exhibiting the 'flight or fight' response to danger (and which results in responses such as galloping off, shying or spooking, or defensive behaviour if the horse is restrained or cornered), it is the endocrine system that maintains the horse in that mode. The nervous system generally works faster than the endocrine system, but the effects of the latter are longer lasting; in the case of the maturing and ageing processes, for example, the effects can last for months or years.

Virtually the entire body is governed by hormones controlling the horse's feelings, behaviour, digestion, growth and development, excretion and other vital functions. Hormones often work together in very complicated chains of events, in cycles or otherwise. Hormone imbalances can cause dysfunction sufficient to kill a horse or simply affect his behaviour or some physical function in some mild way.

GLANDS

Hormone-producing glands are situated at various points of the body (4), although some hormones are in fact produced by organs. The main hormone-producing gland is the pituitary gland, which is situated just beneath the brain; this gland controls the other hormone-producing glands. The pituitary gland itself is controlled by and connected to a small part of the brain called the hypothalamus, which has different centres with many different functions, both autonomic and somatic. It secretes some hormones itself, including releasing and inhibiting factors, which initiate or block other hormonal processes.

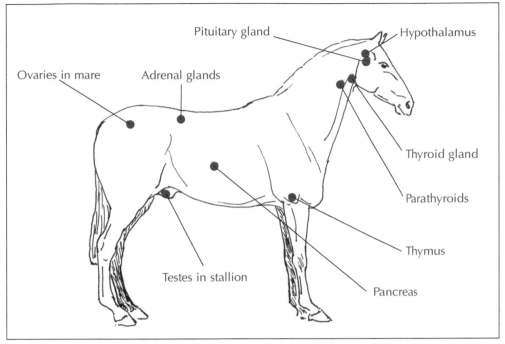

Pituitary gland

Hypothalamus

Ovaries in mare

Adrenal glands

Thyroid gland

Parathyroids

Thymus

Testes in stallion

Pancreas

4 Sites of the major endocrine and exocrine glands.

The glands that secrete the hormones are called endocrine glands or exocrine glands. Endocrine glands secrete hormones for use within the body. They circulate in the blood or lymph and are transported around the body to a particular organ or part distant from the producing gland. Exocrine glands secrete hormones that are concerned with the periphery of the body; for example, sweat and sebaceous glands in the skin; mammary glands involved in milk production; tear glands for keeping the eyes lubricated, clean and healthy; and salivary glands that produce saliva for preparing food for further digestion. Hormones secreted for use locally (near the gland) are sometimes called autacoids.

Other hormonal functions involve sleeping and waking, resting and exercising, lactation, conception, the maintenance of pregnancy, foaling, hunger and thirst, and emotions; indeed, just about every process in the body and every activity the horse undertakes. Probably the two most obvious responses to hormones with which most owners are familiar are the hormonal process responsible for flight in the horse and the oestrus cycle in the mare.

The sequence of events that occurs in these two situations is described below:

- **The flight or fight response** occurs in a horse that has been warned by his nervous system of imminent danger, such as a stalking predator or one that has just started its attack, or a paper bag in the hedge. The horse will usually detect a predator by sight and/or smell and, occasionally, by sound. Electrical impulses shoot along sensory nerves to the CNS, and in a split second others return along motor nerves to the muscles, causing the horse to gallop off. The endocrine system comes into play at once; the pituitary gland sends a chemical message to the adrenal glands near the kidneys to pump the hormone adrenaline into the bloodstream. This produces feelings of excitement and fear, which the horse finds irresistible, and keeps him running, possibly for several minutes. Although the horse may stop running within a very few minutes (or even seconds if he perceives that the danger is over), he may remain excited, alert and restless for hours afterwards. If the horse is unable to run, his response will be to fight and, here again, adrenaline keeps coursing around his body to keep him in survival mode until he no longer perceives a threat.

- **The oestrus cycle of the mare** is a much longer drawn out process, but it can cause behaviour that can be just as concerning to her owner as the flight or fight response. Many mares are accused of being stupid, naughty, uncontrollable (which some may well be), obtuse and all sorts of other insulting descriptions, when in fact they are obeying the feelings induced in them by 'breeding' hormones and are largely powerless to control themselves, whether there is a stallion nearby or not. The cycle occurs over about 21 or 22 days from beginning to end and, while the behaviour of a working mare does affect her performance, understanding and recognizing the various stages of the cycle are also essential for breeders (5). Synthetic hormone administration under veterinary supervision and feeding specific herbal products can control either the cycle or the mare's response to the cycle. In late winter or early spring the cycle starts gearing up but, at this time, it is not regular and conception is unlikely. The pituitary gland releases follicle-stimulating hormone (FSH), a follicle being a fluid-filled sac surrounding an egg in the ovary. This prompts the ovaries to stimulate a few follicles to enlarge and produce oestrogen, the hormone that is responsible for the familiar 'in season' behaviour of squealing, kicking, flirting, splaying the hind legs, producing small amounts of urine frequently and, also, producing mucus from the vulva, 'winking' the vulva and even directing these attentions to humans and other animals in the absence of a stallion. Oestrogen has an inhibitory effect on the pituitary gland, which detects the hormone in the blood flowing through it and then secretes luteinizing hormone (LH), causing one of the follicles to mature, rupture and release its egg. This is the moment of ovulation. A 'yellow body', or corpus luteum, then forms at the site of the ruptured follicle and secretes progesterone (the 'pregnancy hormone'), which takes the mare out of season. Synthetic progesterone is the hormone used to stop competition mares coming into season. If a mare has conceived during her season and is pregnant, she will not come into season again until after foaling. Otherwise, the uterus detects that there is no fertilized egg present and secretes prostaglandin F2α; this instructs the corpus luteum to stop producing progesterone. The corpus luteum regresses and 'dies off', secretion of progesterone ceases and the pituitary gland resumes production of FSH, which begins the cycle all over again. A mare will be 'out of season' for about 16 days and 'in season' for about five days.

These two very different examples of how hormones affect and control a horse should give some idea of their effects. Hormones are extremely powerful substances, without which the horse would not function. Although most hormonal processes go unheeded, some can bring about very noticeable changes in the behaviour of horses.

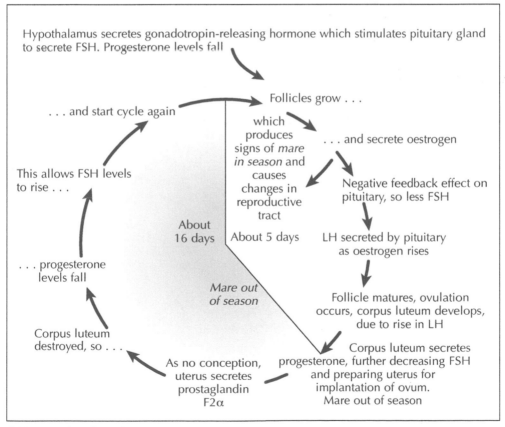

5 Hormonal cycle in the non-pregnant mare.

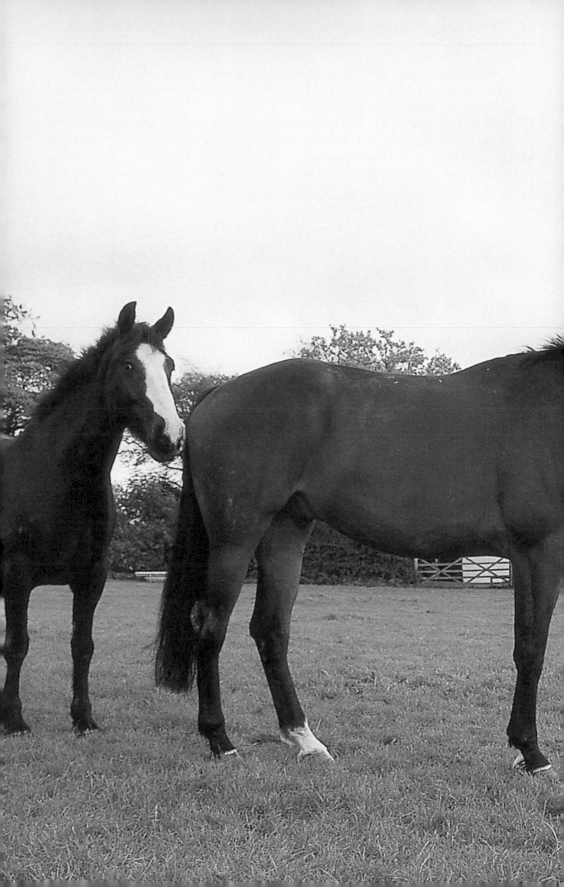

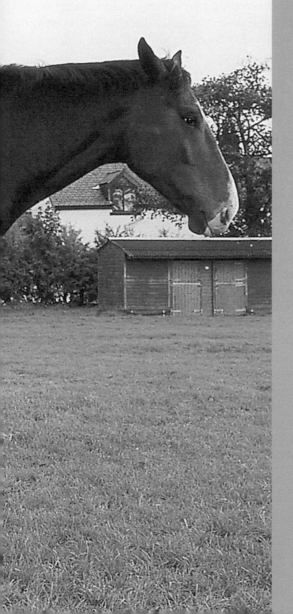

Part 2
Systems of Communication and Information

Part 2 is concerned with the specific basic anatomy and physiology of the five senses as they relate to equine perception and behaviour. It covers how they work, describes our current state of knowledge of them and discusses some of their effects on equine behaviour.

Chapter 3:
The Sense of Smell

Chapter 4:
The Sense of Taste

Chapter 5:
The Sense of Hearing

Chapter 6:
The Sense of Sight

Chapter 7:
The Sense of Touch

Chapter 3
THE SENSE OF SMELL

It may be because humans have such a poor sense of smell, probably one of the worst in the animal kingdom, that we do not realise how much more highly developed is the horse's sense of smell. It may well be almost as powerful and acute as that of a dog, an animal renowned for its ability to follow scent trails, sniff out any substance or recognize and point out to its handler any scent connected with people and other animals, alive or dead. There is no documented record of a horse being specifically trained to do this sort of work, but horses certainly follow scent trails of their own accord. Because horses are so very adaptable and trainable, there seems to be no reason why it would not be possible to utilize this natural ability, although it is much more convenient to use an animal the size of a dog.

NOSTRILS AND NASAL PASSAGES

The nostrils of the horse are very mobile and flexible. They can open ('flare') to a circular shape and close almost to slits to allow for variations in required airflow. Hotblood breeds have larger nostrils than coldblood breeds. This is not only because of the importance to the horse of taking in scents, but also because horses are obligate nasal breathers – they cannot breathe through their mouths. Sniffing in the smells produced by other horses and animals, people, objects, substances and scents left in the air, on the ground and on natural objects such as trees and rocks or on buildings such as stables, usually elicits quite widely opened nostrils.

The nostrils are angled outwards on the muzzle, at ten to and ten past the hour locations. This enables them more easily to take in scents coming from all around their bodies. The nostrils form the outer openings of the nasal passages and they are separated by a septum (partition). The nasal passages contain tightly coiled, thin turbinate bones covered in mucous membrane. This very thin and sensitive tissue, found at several sites in the body, is moist and very vascular (having a good blood supply). It also possesses olfactory (to do with smell) nerve cells, with cilia (tiny hair-like projections) that contain the sensory cells responsible for sensing odours. The coils of the turbinate bones increase the surface area over which odours can spread and be detected by the cells. Odours are actual microscopic, physical particles that dissolve in the moisture of the mucous membranes. The sensory nerve cells in the membranes then send messages to the CNS and the smell is assessed in this way for information, letting the horse know, for example, whether it represents danger, a familiar person or animal, a mare in season, a rival, a different animal or a predator. Smells on objects can apparently last for several days and fresh ones are carried in the air for many minutes or even a few hours on a still day.

JACOBSON'S ORGAN

An important adjunct to the equine olfactory sensory cells is Jacobson's organ, also known as the vomeronasal organ. Its role is to assess odours. It forms two long, thin sacs set on either side of the base of the nasal septum and has nervous connection to the brain. It allows perception of non-volatile material that has been aspirated into the organ when the horse flehmens. Horses use it in the familiar gesture called flehmen to investigate and assess any unusual, intriguing or strange smell (6). The horse will sniff in the odour on a physical carrier (e.g. someone's hands, the ground or a feed bucket) or in the air, raise his or her head and curl up the upper lip, closing off the nostrils and allowing the odour to pass up into the nasal cavity to the organ for closer assessment. Nervous signals pass up the olfactory nerves into the olfactory bulbs at the front of the brain.

Flehmen is not the preserve of stallions. It is performed by all horses, maybe two or three times before they are satisfied with the information they have received.

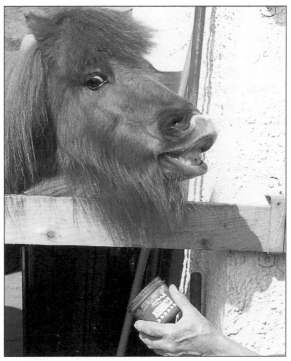

6 Shetland Pony gelding performing the flehmen action in response to a strange smell, in this case the substance in the jar.

THE LIMBIC SYSTEM AND OLFACTION/SENSE OF SMELL

The limbic system in mammals is a group of brain structures concerned with smell or olfaction and certain behaviours to do with emotion and motivation. Two olfactory bulbs are found at the upper end of the olfactory tract on the frontal lobe of each hemisphere of the cerebrum or forebrain. The olfactory nerves have their cell bodies in the mucous membrane of the nasal passages, and pass up, through bony structures, to connect with the olfactory bulbs and from there to the cerebrum.

The olfactory bulbs in the horse are extremely large and their area is increased by their surfaces being convoluted; by comparison, in humans the bulbs are tiny. This gives the reasonable impression that the horse's olfactory system is extremely efficient, well-developed and sophisticated, whereas in humans it is comparatively rudimentary.

SUMMARY

It is hard to imagine a world of scents, such as that experienced by horses, dogs and many other animals, but it is clear that smells are extremely important to them. Horses clearly receive so much more information about their environment from odours than do humans. This includes not only information about the sexual state of other horses both near to them or that have passed by or on the same path as them maybe several days before, but information about the moods and emotions of their herd mates (according to pheromones and hormones released by them), about their feed, about the identity of other horses, animals and people and their environment in general. For these reasons we should start paying more attention to what is one of a horse's most important senses. The practicalities of accommodating and understanding this will be covered in the practical section on management and work in Part 3.

Chapter 4
THE SENSE OF TASTE

The sense of taste is very closely linked neurologically to that of smell. Horses experience taste by means of groups of very small, sensitive papillae or projections, mainly on their tongue but also elsewhere in the mouth (7). Substances that are soluble dissolve into the moistness of the mouth; chewing and mixing with saliva help this process. Receptor cells in the papillae detect the various substances or flavours by means of cilia protruding slightly through the pores in the mucous membrane covering the tongue. Sensory nerve fibres then transmit this information to the gustatory or taste centre in the brain, which, in turn, tells the horse which category of taste the substance falls into. Horses can distinguish between sweet, salty, sour and bitter tastes, and these basic tastes make up in combination all the other tastes. The specialized taste buds able to detect each one are sited on different parts of the tongue.

The mouth, cheeks and tongue contain salivary glands with ducts opening into the mouth along which the saliva passes. The actual feeling of food in the mouth stimulates saliva flow. Saliva is alkaline to neutral on the pH scale (a measure of the degree to which a substance is acidic or alkaline). Saliva contains a digestive enzyme, which starts a little preliminary digestion of starches and sugars, but its main purpose is to soften up food and make it easier to swallow before it reaches the stomach.

Saliva also acts as a buffer against the acidic digestive juices of the stomach. One possible reason why horses that are fed over-large amounts of starchy concentrates and insufficient fibre can develop ulcers is the reduced amount of saliva available to carry out the buffering task. Horses that regularly produce saliva by eating fibre for many hours a day (as the digestive system evolved to function) are apparently less prone to gastric ulcers, although the absence of stress, turning out and a contented life also play a large part. This issue is currently under investigation.

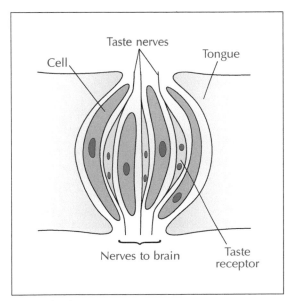

7 Taste bud.

Chapter 5
THE SENSE OF HEARING
(Including Balance)

Sound is one of the three senses horses use to detect the presence of other horses and predators, the other two being smell and vision. Sound consists of air pressure waves of different frequencies stimulating the eardrum. The waves of the lowest frequency detectable by mammals are probably those producing the very low infrasounds used by whales and elephants for information and communication; the highest frequency waves (producing ultrasounds) are used by bats. Horses cannot hear low sounds as well as humans, but they can hear higher sounds. (**NB:** As well as being the organ of sound detection, the ear is also the organ of equilibrium.)

Obviously, the only part of the ear that can be seen is the outer ear (auricle or pinna), which is made of gristly cartilage (8). It is quite large and mobile compared with that of humans. Each ear can be turned by muscles from front to back within an almost 180 degrees semicircle, and the ears can also move independently to pick up sound waves from all around and so pinpoint the direction of sounds. Sound waves are funnelled down to the eardrum or tympanic membrane (9), a thin, delicate membrane that separates and seals off the outer ear from the middle ear.

The middle ear (9) consists of an air-filled cavity behind the eardrum. It is connected to the nasopharynx d(upper nose and throat area) by the auditory tube, which enables the air pressure on the inner ear side of the eardrum to be maintained equal to that on its outer ear surface. There are three ossicles or small bones forming a chain across the middle ear from the eardrum to the window of the inner ear (also called the labyrinth). These transmit the sound waves. They are called the malleus (hammer), incus (anvil) and stirrup (stapes) because of their function or shape. The hammer is in contact with the eardrum so, when the latter vibrates, having been stimulated by sound waves, the hammer in turn vibrates on the adjacent anvil. The vibrations in turn travel from the other end of the anvil to the stirrup, which passes them on into the inner ear. Very small muscles are attached to these ossicles. They contract when

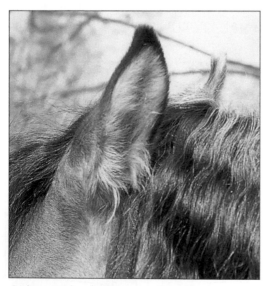

8 The outside of the ear, or pinna. The protective hairs growing in it are to help prevent foreign bodies falling down inside the ear. They should not be trimmed out, only neatened at the edges and base where they protrude beyond the edges of the ear.

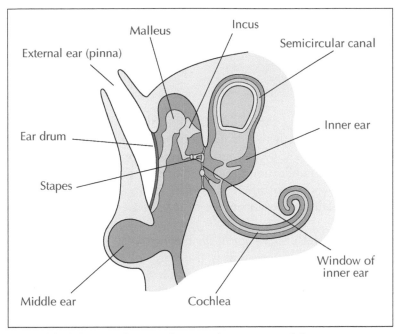

9 Simplified diagram showing the complex structure of the ear.

loud or piercing sound vibrations hit the eardrum, to some degree protecting the eardrum and the inner ear from injury.

The inner ear (9) is just inside the skull and contains fluid-filled tubes concerned with hearing and equilibrium or balance. One such tube is a curled structure called the cochlea. The cochlea contains sensitive hairs and the sensory nerve, which transmits the electrical impulses stimulated by the sound waves to the brain. Sound waves can pass through air, fluid and solids, so they travel down the ossicles into the inner ear. The vibrations of the stapes against the window of the inner ear set the fluid in the inner ear in motion. This is picked up by the cochlea, and sensory nervous impulses then send the message to the auditory centre in the brain.

Above the cochlea are the three semicircular canals. These are set at right angles to each other in three dimensions, two being vertical and one horizontal. The canals are essential for balance and the detection of movement, and they contain a fluid called endolymph. The canals are enlarged at their ends (the ampullae). Sense organs in the ampullae contain sensory hairs. When the horse moves his head even a little, the fluid in the canal lying in the plane of that movement presses against the sensory hairs on the nerves in the ampullae. These detect the direction of the movement, initiating nerve impulses, which then travel to the brain. This is how the brain detects the horse's equilibrium and, in extreme movements and some disorders, can produce a feeling of giddiness.

Chapter 6
THE SENSE OF SIGHT

The sense of sight of horses is the sense least like that of humans. Despite considerable research, there is still much that is not known about the sense of sight in horses. However, our state of knowledge has progressed considerably during the decade preceding the date of publication of this book to the point where it is at least known that horses see the world very differently from the way it is seen by humans. This goes a long way to explaining the sometimes strange and erratic behaviour displayed by horses.

The mammalian eyeball develops in the embryo as an extension of the brain. It is a very delicate and sensitive organ; it is also very vulnerable despite being protected by the bones of the orbital cavity in the skull. Some protection is offered by the conjunctiva, a moist, delicate, transparent membrane that covers the surface of the eye as far as the junction with the cornea (the transparent front of the eye). The eyelashes (which in horses, unlike humans, are only on the upper lids) also give some protection. Tears from the lacrimal (tear) glands constantly wash the eye, keeping it moist and comfortable and helping to remove foreign bodies. As it has no blood supply, the cornea receives much of its nourishment from gases in the air and from the edge of the eye and the inside of the eye. It is the fastest tissue in the body to heal, and can actually be watched doing so under magnification.

As a classic prey animal, the horse has its eyes set out to the sides of the head, giving him an almost all-round view (about 330 degrees) to check for predators. The eyeball is an oblate spheroid (a slightly more than flattened sphere, in this case flattened from front to back) (10), and it is constructed of three layers. There is a strong, white, opaque, outer layer consisting of connective tissue, called the sclera, of which the transparent cornea is a continuation. The middle layer is the choroid, which has a good blood supply, and the third layer is the retina, the light-sensitive 'screen' onto which images are projected. The retina contains specialized sensory nerve cells, known because of their different shapes as rods and cones. Rods work well in dim light and can interact with other cells in the retina in detecting movement rather than sharp detail. Cones are able to detect colour and better detail in brighter light, but not so sharply as in humans.

To assist in acquiring as much light as possible in dim light situations, the horse has one of the largest eyes relative to body size in the animal world. There is also a light reflective layer beneath the upper half of the retina called the tapetum, as in other nocturnal animals. This bounces back any light not absorbed by the cells, giving them a second chance to capture the photons (light particles) entering the eye, but this is at the expense of some clarity. The tapetum accounts for the reflection of the eyes of nocturnal animals if you shine a torch onto them at night or capture them in certain circumstances with flash photography, if the animal is looking directly at the light source.

Towards the bottom of the retina is a small blind spot (not covered by the light sensitive retina), of which the horse is not aware. This is the point where the optic nerve joins the eye, its purpose being to transmit nerve impulses from the retina to the visual centre of the brain. The nerves from the rods and cones are gathered together in this one main nerve.

The lens is suspended by small, rather weak muscles, so the horse has poor accommodation or ability to focus onto near objects by means of the lens. Behind the cornea and in front of the lens is the iris, a circular, usually brown-coloured band of tissue with a horizontal oval hole in the middle (the pupil). It can widen or narrow to adjust the amount of light entering the eye. On the lower edge of the upper part of the iris, immediately above the pupil, are the corpora nigra (granula iridica), or black bodies, which act as inbuilt sunshades. Because of their location, they also restrict upward vision and are probably instrumental in creating the famous 'blind spot' that the horse has in an upward direction immediately in front of the face for a distance of something less than six feet.

The area between the lens and the cornea is filled with a watery fluid called aqueous humour, which provides some nourishment for the lens and cornea and helps to maintain the pressure inside this part of the eyeball and, so, the optical integrity of the structure. The area between the lens and the retina is filled with a more gel-like fluid called vitreous humour, which has similar purposes.

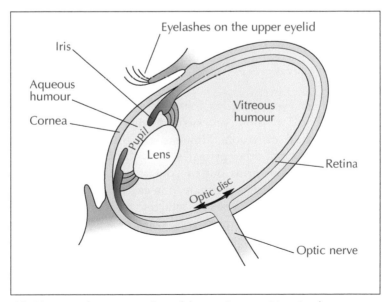

10 Diagram of a cross-section of the equine eye. Note its shape, which is much less spherical than the human eye.

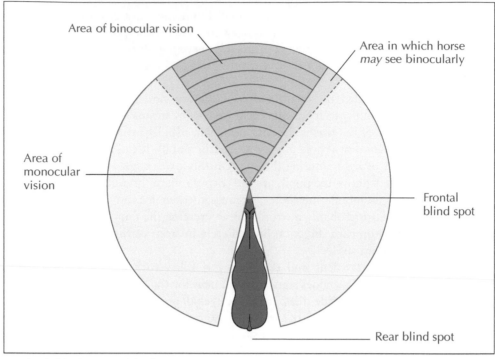

11 The field of vision of the horse.

Predators have their eyes set facing forwards so that they can concentrate with both eyes (called 'binocular vision', *bi* = two) on what they are hunting. This restricts the extent of their field of vision. Humans are mainly predators and so have predator's eyes. Humans and other primates see within a circular area mainly ahead of them. If you stretch your arms out to your sides and look straight ahead you cannot see them. However, being a primate, you can see very sharply (with excellent 'acuity', given normal to good eyesight) straight in front of you and less clearly around the central sharp area, your peripheral vision area. (Dogs and cats do not have as good acuity as humans, which is surprising considering that both these species are effective predators. This is because primates, including humans, have a macula, which is the area of the retina giving this very sharp central area of vision, and carnivores do not have anything nearly as well developed.)

The area of vision to the sides, seen with only one eye, is the monocular vision (*mono* = one) area. In the horse this extends almost right around the body so that he can detect movement, such as a possible predator (**11**). The horse's area of binocular vision comprises about 60–70 degrees in front of his head.

A high level of acuity exists in primates because only they have a macula, with a small pit or depression (the fovea) in the central area of the retina. Cone cells only are concentrated in the fovea, making high acuity detail and good colour vision possible, from red to violet in the spectrum. Primate retinas have a high ratio of cones to rods in areas of the retina other than the fovea (the peripheral vision area), but vision in these areas is not so acute; therefore, primates (including humans) can detect movement 'out of the corner of their eye' and can tell that objects are there, but may well not know just what they are. Because the fovea of primates has no rods, humans also have the disadvantage of not seeing at all clearly in low-light conditions.

The macula of the equine retina has more rods than cones. This means that horses cannot see as 'sharply' or 'clearly' as humans. This is exacerbated by the fact that they have poor accommodation (i.e. they cannot alter the shape of their lens with their ciliary muscles to bring close-up objects into focus, as can be done in humans). Therefore, horses have only reasonably good acuity and the lack of cones also means that they see less well than humans in bright light, but better in the dark. Actual darkness hampers any creature's vision, as the reflection of light onto the retina is key to the stimulation of the photoreceptors (the rods and cones) in the retina.

The field of vision of horses consists of a horizontal band of their best acuity in comparison with the circular spot of best acuity found in humans. This is due to a 'visual streak' just below the equator of the retina. Horses can see almost all around them in a strip in which their acuity is quite good and is better than in the area above and below, but not so acute as that produced by the human fovea. Independent of the shape of the high-acuity region, both humans and horses may experience a wider field.

The horse's eye does not move far or easily in its bony socket (unlike the eye of humans) and this characteristic, plus the poor accommodation and the visual streak, means that the horse needs to move his head around, up and down and from side to side a good deal in order to bring objects onto the visual streak and obtain the best view possible. It is not a case of the horse having to focus objects onto a ramp-shaped retina, as was previously thought, but of him needing to manoeuvre his head and, therefore, his eyes and visual streaks into the best position to capture the image he is trying to look at.

As a grazing animal, it is important for the horse to be able to see down to the ground clearly when his head is lowered and to identify plants to eat. This is what the function and placement of his eyes enable him to do. Horses can also see where they are putting their feet at slower gaits when the head is slightly flexed at the poll. The binocular area is therefore directed down the front of the face. In order to see ahead the horse must lift his head and point his muzzle towards where he wants to go, or is being asked by his rider or driver to go, something that is often denied to domestic horses during work because of the 'held-in' head position so often demanded.

Horses, because of their fairly wide area of binocular vision, can assess quite accurately the distance they are from objects. Therefore, they have little trouble 'seeing a stride' when jumping, for example, if allowed to do so by their riders. Close objects can be brought more clearly into view onto the visual streak (bearing in mind the poor accommodation ability of the lens in the eye) if the horse is allowed to slightly tilt and lower his head, depending on the position of the object, whether it is food on the ground or something in his way or which he wants to investigate. The eyes of a horse evolved to be long-sighted, as would be expected in a prey animal that often has to run for its life.

Despite having monocular vision almost all around them, horses do not have eyes like a chameleon (i.e. moving independently all around their bodies). However, it is known that horses can make use of the different views coming in from the two eyes, combining them in a process called stereopsis (but only in the binocular visual field). There would seem little point in evolution having created in them this type of vision if they could not do so. It is another aid to recognizing predators in the forms of shape and movement. It seems that horses have great difficulty in recognizing completely stationary objects, people and animals.

Colour vision has long been an old chestnut in conversation about horses. Many lay horse enthusiasts have maintained for generations that horses and other animals are colour-blind, seeing things only in tones of black, grey and white, and the equestrian press frequently used to publish letters from readers on this topic. It is noticeable that this type of correspondence no longer seems to appear, so perhaps the results of scientific research have filtered through to the horse world in general.

The range of six colours humans can see is what most people were taught in physics at school – red, orange, yellow, green, blue and violet. There is a familiar mnemonic to help us remember these colours – Richard Of York Gave Battle In Vain. Because there is a letter I in there, many people include the composite colour of indigo, but scientists tend not to include it in the spectrum as a 'true' colour. However, looking through a spectrometer or at a diamond in bright light is fascinating, and many other wonderful colours (e.g. turquoise, lavender, brown, peach and cerise) can be seen. These additional colours are made up from amalgamations of the basic six colours.

The electromagnetic spectrum goes: x-rays/gamma rays; ultraviolet; violet; blue; green; yellow; orange; red; far red; infrared; microwaves; and radio waves. The red end of the spectrum is carried by longer light waves and the blue end by shorter ones.

It appears from recent scientific research that horses, along with dogs and cats, are dichromats (*di* = two), having two types of cones that differ in the spectrum of wavelengths over which they absorb, thus enabling them to distinguish colours in two ranges from the spectrum – the red/orange part and the blue/purple part of the spectrum, and colours containing these in their make-up. Humans are trichromats (*tri* = three) and so are able to see colours in the yellow/green area of the spectrum as well. Work on equine colour vision continues, however, both in formal scientific studies and in informal situations. Some observers feel that horses can see colours in the middle part of the human visual spectrum, maybe at the expense of some red or violet colours. The luminance or brightness of a colour (the 'shininess', for instance) can also affect the appearance of colours.

Birds, some fish and insects can see into the ultraviolet spectrum, some fish can see into the far red spectrum and some reptiles can see microwaves. Because light waves are capable of stimulating the different types of cones in an animal's retina, colour (and, it could be said, sight itself) is a subjective experience depending not only on the type of cone cells possessed by an individual creature, but also on the species to which it belongs.

In humans sight has evolved as their most important sense. We may well wonder how horses cope with having such different (some would say much poorer) vision from us, but their senses of hearing and, particularly, smell are 'better' than ours and they rely on them greatly in the daily battle of wits with predators in their natural or feral environments.

The whole structure and function of the horse's eye are further indicators of an animal that has evolved to live in wide open spaces, to detect prey and to operate optimally in dim light conditions. Horses cannot see well in bright light and no creature can see in total darkness. The horse probably sees visual detail in general slightly better than we can see within our peripheral vision. Their three-dimensional vision is not as good as ours. As would be expected in a prey animal, they can detect moving objects much more accurately than humans. Left to organize their own lives, which few domestic horses are, horses are most active at dawn and dusk and their vision must have something to do with this, as this is when they can see optimally, which is, at the best of times, rather indistinctly compared with humans.

Chapter 7
THE SENSE OF TOUCH

The skin (**12**) is the main covering of the horse's body, although two related structures, horn and hair, are very similar to it. Together they are called the common integument. They consist of a fibrous, hardened protein substance called keratin, which, in use, flakes off or is worn away, although horn often needs trimming. Skin is mainly covered by hair, which is a mammalian characteristic, although the terms 'hair' or 'hair-like' are used to describe other structures such as cilia.

Horn is found around the feet and also in the chestnuts on the insides of the legs, and it forms the ergots on the points of the fetlocks. Although it is basically 'dead' (insensitive, having no nerves or blood supply), horses can certainly sense pressure or vibrations through horn (e.g. when having shoes hammered on or having hooves squeezed with hoof testers to diagnose pain in the feet) and, quite possibly, through the ground. (An incident was reported in *Equine Behaviour* concerning a shod horse who would not be turned out in a particular field where, it was later discovered, there was a faulty electric cable running under the ground. His companions were unshod and were unaffected.)

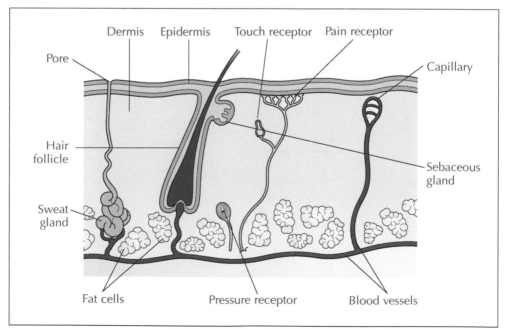

12 Basic diagram of the structures in the skin.

The outermost layer of the skin (the epidermis) is similar to horn, having no nerves or blood supply, but it is very thin and easily transmits as light a touch as an irritating fly, never mind a biting one. Although the skin has five layers, for practical purposes it is useful to think of two main ones: the epidermis and the sensitive, vascular (having a blood supply) dermis beneath it. It is the dermis that contains the microscopic blood capillaries, the sweat glands, the sebaceous (oil) glands, the hair follicles and roots and the little erector muscles associated with them, and also the nerve endings or receptors that sense pain (nociceptors), pressure, touch and vibration (mechanoreceptors) and temperature (thermoreceptors) and that are distributed variably in the body. The skin's mass is made up of cells, collagen (a protein substance), elastin (which gives it its suppleness and flexibility) and other fibres.

Under the skin is a subcutaneous layer where fat is normally stored as an insulator. The subcutaneous layer consists mainly of loose, fibrous connective tissue. This enables one to slide the skin under the flat of one's hand over the structures beneath. Doing this over the ribcage is a test of skin and health condition.

From the description above it is clear that the skin is a vital organ, which provides a life-saving envelope around the body. It is the largest organ of the body and is not only crucial to life, but is a reflector of the horse's state of health and well-being. For the purposes of this book, however, our interest is in the fact that the skin contains many nervous receptors that transmit messages along sensory nerves to the CNS and so play an important role in informing the horse of what is happening to him.

SIMPLIFIED STRUCTURE AND FUNCTION OF NERVES

Vertebrates have highly developed nervous systems and the horse is just as sensitive to touch as humans and, some believe, more so. Neurones (or nerve cells) are organized into nerves and collections of nerve cell bodies (ganglions), which form a network of nerves all around the body.

The cell bodies have a nucleus, which is the site of transcription of DNA into an RNA message that leaves the nucleus and is translated into proteins in the cytoplasm. The cell bodies also have two or more appendages. These may be very short and branching (called dendrites) and they receive and send sensory messages towards the ganglion/cell body. Cell bodies also have a single, longer fibre (the axon), which can be up to several metres long in large animals and which transmits messages away from the cell body to other nerves. The ends, again, are branched.

Between two neurones at the nerve endings, where they almost meet, is a small junction or gap called a synapse. At the synapse, the impulse or message causes release of a neurotransmitter, a chemical that diffuses across the gap and binds to receptors on the second neurone, causing it to fire off a new impulse. In this way, impulses are transferred from one neurone to another and messages are sent along a chain of sensory nerves to the CNS, which, similarly, sends messages back down motor ('action') nerves to the nerve endings in the muscles and/or glands.

When the nerve endings are stimulated several times in rapid succession, their response can become 'worn out' for a while and may, in a mild case, need several seconds to resume normal function. It is also possible for repeated overstimulation to temporarily destroy their response. An example of this is when a vet thumps a particular spot three or four times before inserting a needle to give an injection; the horse hardly feels the needle going in. It is sometimes suggested that riders who give a leg aid or who even kick at every stride effectively 'deaden' the horse's response to the stimulus, and also that those who ride with a constant, harsh contact are actually creating a 'dead' or hard mouth in their horse, which may become permanent.

The lack of response to constant leg contact may be behavioural, due to the horse coming to regard the pressure as 'white noise', and the permanent changes in hard mouths may also be behavioural (due to the plasticity of synapses in the CNS) or physical (real callous formation) or perhaps a combination of both.

REFLEXES

Another form of nervous transmission is the reflex. A reflex is described as an involuntary reaction to a stimulus (i.e. it does not need the intervention of conscious thought). This means that the horse does not have to think about his response; his nervous system responds for him. Examples of reflex actions are blinking, coughing, sneezing, shivering, swallowing, moving away from sudden pain, twitching muscles to remove irritating insects or turning round when its name is called.

Reflex actions take place by means of a reflex arc. A reflex arc is the simplest functional unit of the nervous system, consisting of an afferent or sensory receptor transmitting messages/nervous impulses along its nerve axon to the CNS, usually the spinal cord. Here, the messages are passed via interneurones or relay neurones to an efferent or motor neurone and thence to an effector organ (a gland or muscle that carries out the 'effect' of the messages) to instruct it to make an appropriate response. Therefore, the arc is a circuit or pathway consisting of receptor, sensory nerve, CNS, motor nerve and effector.

It is argued by some scientists that once a horse's response to an aid or any other stimulus becomes habitual, it will respond without thinking (i.e. reflexively), because horses are claimed by them to be creatures of habit and instinct rather than thought; however, many practical horsemen and women would deny this. Riders all know that, to a large degree, the horse can certainly decide or control whether or not he responds to a nervous impulse in the form of an aid or command and just what response he will give. For example, in response to a hand or leg aid on his side, he can decide whether or not to move and how to move.

Stimuli such as aids and commands are termed conditioned reflexes because the horse is conditioned by learning and repetition to respond to them. New pathways and junctions between nerve endings actually develop within the nervous system so that once the habit is developed, the horse responds automatically whenever the appropriate stimulus occurs. Therefore, theoretically, not only can desired responses to the aids become reflex actions, but they can also become unwanted actions such as shying at general or specific things that move and elicit a 'startle' response, or shying in one particular place. The more something happens the more likely is the horse to respond reflexively and reliably, whether you want him to or not. Fortunately, undesirable conditioned reflexes can be overridden by new training and learning experiences.

SUMMARY

The horse's sense of touch is so exquisitely sensitive that we really should pay more regard to it when we have anything to do with our horses. It is fairly easy for humans to try to put right anything that is irritating or hurting them or making them feel uncomfortable due to extremes of temperature, or to give themselves relief or pleasure by scratching or rubbing themselves or having a skilled massage. We make it much more difficult for our horses to do the same. Free horses wearing no equipment and with access to company and to shelter in inclement weather, both hot and cold, are in the same position as we always are. A lot of the time, though, they are made uncomfortable due to lack of shelter from insects or weather; clothing that is uncomfortable, sometimes very uncomfortable, and worn for nearly all of the time; an inability to attend to their own bodies beneath that clothing or to remove it; lack of access to other horses for mutual grooming or of somewhere to rub themselves; an inability to control the air quality and ventilation in their stables; and a lack of acceptable facilities in which to roll such as adequate space or a surface they consider suitable.

Rough handling such as from the ground, under the saddle or in harness can also be very upsetting and frightening for many horses. Sadly, some people today often purposely inflict pain on these sensitive animals, maybe through harsh use of the bit, reins and spurs or in the form of a beating with a whip, often under the guise of correction or punishment for perceived misdemeanours – so-called discipline – but also because they lose self-control and take it out on their horses. Some of the training techniques used throughout the horse world can surely be regarded as abusive when they are considered along with a better understanding of the horse's very sensitive body and how his sense of touch and, of course, his other senses, affect his mind.

More attention to the horse's sense of touch and its effects on his mind, body and welfare would improve the lot of most horses.

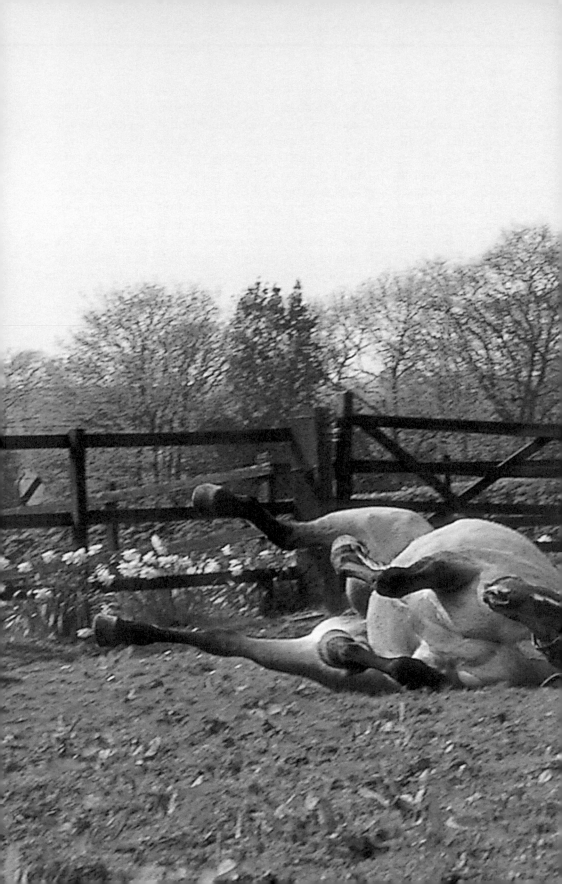

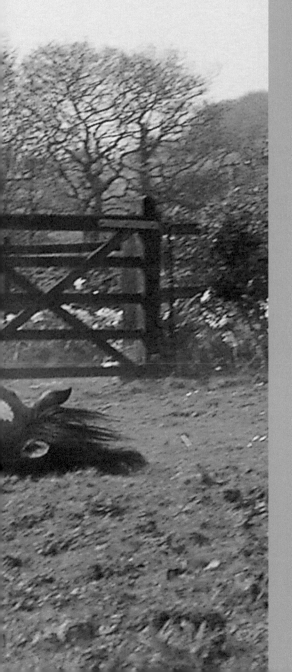

Part 3
Management and Work

This is the largest and most practical part of the book, bringing together the functioning of the senses and how they relate to the ways in which we should manage, care for and work horses and ponies. Many examples and anecdotes from real life are given to illustrate points made to inform and, I hope, entertain readers.

Chapter 8:
The Sense of Smell

Chapter 9:
The Sense of Taste

Chapter 10:
The Sense of Hearing

Chapter 11:
The Sense of Sight

Chapter 12:
The Sense of Touch

Chapter 8
THE SENSE OF SMELL

The sense of smell is probably the one most underrated by riders and carers of horses. This is possibly because the sense of smell in humans is so rudimentary in comparison and there is a tendency to overlook how important most animals' sense of smell is to them.

A horse uses his sense of smell all the time, rather in the way that a dog does (**13, 14**). He smells everyone who comes near him (**15**); he can smell and recognize people from many yards away; he uses smell to identify other animals, whether horses or other species, including predatory ones; he uses his sense of smell to identify and select grasses and other plants plus the feed (**16**) and water offered to him; and he can smell if other horses have been where he has been and even when and the state they were in.

Because horses have less distinct vision than people, they use smell, along with hearing, a great deal in identification. An owner or other attendant who sees a particular horse or horses regularly may not think it important how he or she smells, but imagine how confusing it must be for a horse to be dealt with by people whose smell frequently changes. Their equine companions will smell largely the same all the time, other than mares or fillies in oestrus/season; however, a horse understands this and he can rely on familiar horses smelling more or less the same all the time. Horses realize that their normal smell changes fairly slowly according to their hormonal state, and this applies to stallions as well as to mares. Humans, however, may change their toiletries, change the products in which they wash their clothes, use a different dry-cleaner for certain clothes or wear different fabrics, which smell differently. Our smell will also change slightly if we have touched other people or animals; shaking hands with someone or stroking a dog or cat or another horse, for example, will result in a different smell on our hands and maybe our clothes.

OH, IT'S YOU – OR IS IT?
Many years ago, when I had recently bought my much loved first horse, I was going out in the evening to a party held near his livery yard. I thought this was a good chance to pay him an extra visit and show him off to my date, so I called in on the way, all freshly bathed, shampooed, made up, perfumed and wearing completely different clothes from the ones I wore for 'horsing around'. We also arrived in my date's car rather than my father's, which I always used, so the engine sound gave the horse no warning. When the horse saw me clicking along the apron in my high heels and glad rags, he took one glance and, unusually, turned back inside to his hay. He did not recognize my appearance and, when I reached his box and spoke to him, he turned to come and stopped halfway across, looking uncertain and confused. Not only did I look different, I smelled different, too, and he only recognized me from my voice.

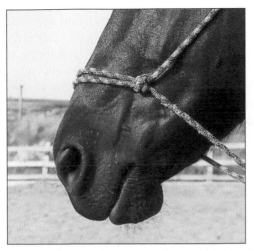 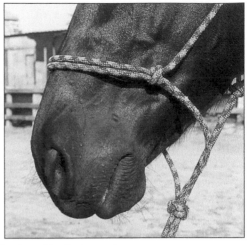

13, 14 (13) Nostrils open in a horse. (14) Nostrils closed in the same horse.

15 Horses use their sense of smell to investigate just about anything, including people.

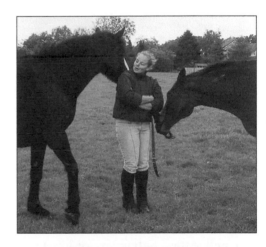

16 Investigating possible food (an onion).

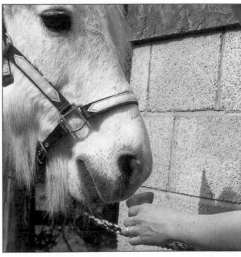

He spent the whole of this short visit, even after he accepted that it was me, smelling me up and down with great interest. At the end of the visit, I walked away down the apron again, turned at the end, and he was watching me from his box as if trying to work out these mixed messages he had received. Therefore, it is sensible, when associating with horses, to always use the same day-to-day toiletries, within reason. It has been suggested that deodorants, talc, scent, perfumed soaps, after-shave or anything similar should not be used at all when around horses, but products used regularly do become a part of our smell and mingle with our individual body scent, and so form 'our' smell.

I once kept my horse in the same yard as a good friend and I used to ride his horses, too, when he could not be there. I remember borrowing a coat of his from the tack room on a particularly cold day and my own horse and his two were all quite confused by this. They all clearly knew who I was and I smelled of the familiar me to some extent, but there was also an undeniable smell of my friend coming from the coat. What on earth was happening? My own horse followed me around his box sniffing first of all my face and neck and then my friend's coat, then me again; however, my friend's horses sniffed only his coat. Once aboard, they seemed to forget all about their 'aromatic confusion' and behaved as normal when ridden. Each time I returned from a ride they reverted to sniffing the coat until I took it off, and then behaved normally.

Smell is a horse's second line of enquiry after vision when checking on the identity or condition of others. A normal horse greeting is a nostril-to-nostril exchange of breath, which not only identifies the individuals to each other but tells them what the other has been eating. Horses also sometimes smell each other's chestnuts (17), which apparently have a very individual smell; old nagsmen often used to peel off a bit of chestnut and rub it on their hands to encourage the horse to accept them. This practice also works for getting horses used to new equipment. Smells or pheromones from other parts of the body, particularly the groin and tail area but also other areas, tell others what state a horse is in (e.g. whether he is nervous or frightened or, on the other hand, calm; what sex the horse is; his state of health; and even, some say, his age and status). Submissive or low-ranking horses may be more anxious all the time and so give off pheromones or smells associated with low levels of fear. Feral horses may be able to identify what area a strange horse lives in just from the smell of the food on his breath, which may be different from that in his own home area.

Sweat enhances a horse's overall smell. It varies between the sweat produced because of work and the excretion of waste products, sweating because of fear or sweating because the horse needs to cool down. Horses sweat most of the time. Owners only notice it when the amount produced is significant enough to wet the coat hair before it has a chance to evaporate into the surrounding air, or if the air is already humid and evaporation is hardly possible. Horses probably have the highest sweating rate of all animals, including humans; in contrast, dogs only sweat through their paws.

SMELLING TROUBLE

My own horse also illustrated clearly what many owners already know – horses can smell a vet or a farrier a mile away, figuratively speaking. He once needed to have a course of moderately painful injections and had started becoming upset when the vet arrived. On the last day of his course a new vet arrived in a different car, but the aroma surrounding him must have been just the same (a general medical-type smell perhaps), because as soon as the vet stepped out of his car a few yards away the horse sniffed the air, retreated to the back of his box and started tossing his head. This was his way of expressing anxiety.

Another horse I owned always played up when I approached him with a particular product my vet had prescribed to treat a troublesome and very sore leg injury, presumably because he associated its particular smell with something stressful and unpleasant about to happen.

Horses may also identify others from the smell of their rugs because they, too, become impregnated with the smell of their normal wearer. For hygiene reasons, it is advised that clothing is not changed from horse to horse, but occasionally it may be necessary to borrow and this can cause an 'identity crisis' by confusing the horse's companions. Horses can, in cases like this, smell the rightful owner of the rug and also smell the parts of the wearer not covered by it, become confused and, as horses often do when uncertain or worried, either avoid the situation (i.e. the horse) completely or actually attack him because they cannot work out who he is or simply because he represents something confusing and incomprehensible.

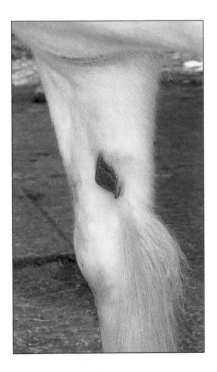

17 The horny chestnuts on the insides of horses' and ponies' legs smell quite strongly. They can also be used for visual identification, like a person's fingerprints, as they are all different.

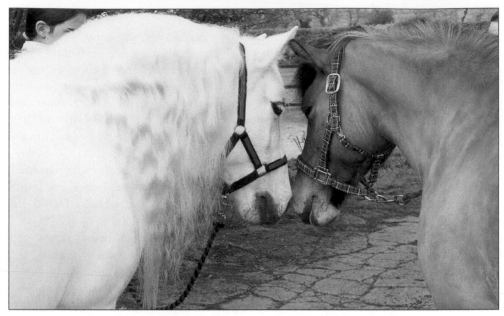

18 Normal horse to horse greeting.

Smell is also extremely important to horses in social exchanges, particularly with introductions. Horses new to each other will approach head to head, sometimes slightly sideways, and exchange breath via their nostrils (18). They sniff in each other's smell, then usually expel the air quite forcibly down the nostrils, snorting to clear their nasal passages (and, presumably, Jacobson's organ) ready for another dose of the new horse's personal identifying signature. Many people try to stop horses doing this or only allow it for a very brief time because it is often accompanied by squealing and possibly striking out or, occasionally, by a turn and the threat of a kick. Naturally, no one wants their horse to be injured, but if the horses are kept more or less side to side and the handlers, if any, stay on the outsides of the pair, and they are walked about together, there is, in my experience, not a problem. An ideal way to introduce two strange horses is to ride them out together (19), stand or walk them side by side and let them look at and smell each other. After this it should be fine to turn them out together.

Where strange horses are turned free together, it should be in as large and safe a paddock as possible so that if there are antisocial reactions, one horse has plenty of room to escape from the other (20). They will be seen to approach as described and exchange breath via the nostrils, first one then the other. Their mouths may or may not be open. A particularly submissive or young animal may tap his or her front teeth together at the other one with an extended muzzle (21), which is a horse's way of saying 'I recognize that you might hurt me, but please do not.'

19 After the initial meeting, a good way to let ponies get to know each other is to hack them out together.

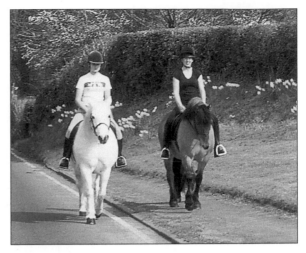

20 This pony is playing a potentially dangerous game, approaching the horse from behind. In some company this could result in a kick from the horse. The horse indicates by his ear position and his eyes that he knows that the pony is there and does not plan to do anything about it. In fact, these two know each other well.

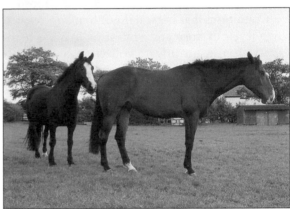

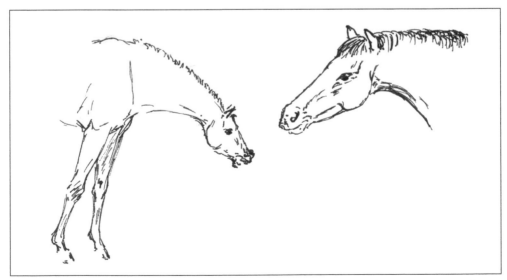

21 The distinctive action of 'snapping' is used by submissive or young horses to communicate a non-threatening attitude.

Horses may not like to wear equipment belonging to and smelling of another horse, even if they are friendly with that horse. When clothing is laundered and, therefore, smells different, horses often smell it, either intently or at least by making an olfactory note of it as it is put on them. They presumably like their own clothing and equipment to smell of themselves, and this certainly seems to be the case with their stables and bedding.

Many owners complain that a horse will nearly always either stale (urinate) or do a dropping (defecate) on fresh bedding. Although horses are said not to be territorial, urine and faeces are used all the time as markers of a herd's territory. At liberty, horses normally avoid their own urine and droppings, so it does not seem accurate in these circumstances to say that they are marking the new bedding with their own smell. However, as stabled horses, even though they cannot normally touch each other, are kept closer together and so more crowded than in nature, this may be a way of declaring personal space, brought on by the stress of confinement and close neighbours, which may not be of their choosing.

Conditions that horses, if not humans, regard as overcrowded are known to create high levels of stress and aggression in horse herds, as do overlarge groups. During the 1980s I visited a private collection of Przewalski horses to write an article about them. There was one stallion and four mares plus their foals on about twelve acres (five hectares) of land. Young horses were removed at puberty, as would often happen in the wild, and sent to reintroduction and conservation schemes around the world. The owner had tried to introduce two other adult mares, one at a time, but the stallion, although not normally aggressive, had killed them both (by disembowelling them if I remember correctly). The owner believed the stallion felt that there was only enough space for his present herd size. Food availability was not an issue. Interestingly, there were also two collections of zebras (Grevy's and plains zebras) on this estate, both of which were much more approachable than the Przewalski horses.

Memories in humans are often evoked by scents (they can take you back years) and I am sure that this happens in horses. It certainly happens in dogs. I sponsor a dog with a canine charity whose first owner was a violent alcoholic. The dog, now nine years old, cannot bear the smell of alcohol, smoke or general domestic smells such as cooking and cleaning fluids because he associates them with a home environment (he cannot be re-homed) and being abused. It may well be that this association of smells is just that (i.e. a trigger or link between a smell and pain), but equally, actual memory could just as easily play a part. My own dog backs away if a man enters the house and I believe that this is because a male social worker came and took her away from her first family, who could not cope with her.

It is quite possible that some of the apparently strange and inexplicable behaviour patterns horses show could well be a reaction to memories triggered by certain smells.

PROFESSIONAL BEHAVIOUR

When horses are working in some branch of show business (e.g. horse theatre, circus, displays) they are often trained to do their droppings before doing their act because audiences, most members of which are not experienced with horses, find it embarrassing or amusing for a horse to do droppings during a performance. It is also inconvenient for the people involved to have to work around them and for stagehands to have to remove them after their particular 'spot'. These horses are trained by having a pile of their own or the droppings of some subordinate horse placed in a particular spot (a specific site being chosen and kept to for each different venue), then each horse in upward rank order being taken to the pile, allowed to smell it and do their own droppings on top of it. As most such horses are stallions, they are usually very ready to try to mask the smell of the previous horse. As the horse is doing his droppings in this way, a vocal command will be chosen and subsequently used so that the horse comes to associate that word with doing a dropping, and will often do so on command in future.

Horses can also be taught to stale on command before exercise or travelling; for example, if a horse is taught to associate staling with a particular word or whistle, then he will stale whenever he hears this word or whistle. I have easily taught my own horses to do this, and dogs commonly urinate at a specific request from their owners.

A PLACE OF HIS OWN

It must be very unsettling for horses to be regularly moved around within their yard into boxes used by other horses, as happens in some establishments. Other reasons apart, they can obviously smell that this is not 'their' bit of territory and, particularly if the previous occupant was a horse with which they do not get on, it can be quite worrying for them, even if the previous horse left months earlier. Whenever I have changed livery yards, I have done my best to completely clear out the box allocated to my horse and have cleaned the floor and as far up the walls as I could with a horse-friendly disinfectant, to try to remove other equine smells at least.

It is noticeable that new horses in a yard often seem to do more droppings and to stale more, and to leave their deposits all around their new box. This may be because they are on edge and have not settled in, or because they sense that their immediate neighbours are not particularly friendly, but it could also be because they are trying to mask the smell, even an old smell, of the previous occupant and impregnate the box with their own smells. After a few days or weeks, many horses choose particular parts of their stables to do their droppings; they will also choose particular places to stale if the box is big enough to allow male horses a choice.

I once had a very self-possessed old Thoroughbred mare who settled immediately into a yard I moved her to, choosing her dunging and staling area at once, virtually ignoring her neighbours and deciding within days whom she would allow to attend her. The box had been thoroughly cleaned before putting her new bedding down and this may have helped her to settle. The first thing she did on arrival was smell the bedding, check the view out of the back window and the positions of the water and haylage, and then started eating. She neither dunged nor staled for about an hour.

With many horses moving yards is a very different story and some take it quite badly. My friend's horse, very much a one-person horse, was moved to a different livery yard and was still very unsettled after more than a fortnight. A therapist said that she felt the horse would benefit by my friend leaving her jacket with him at night times, and told her not to wash the jacket first. She did this and every morning afterwards she found it on the bedding and well flattened. The horse obviously took the jacket off the door and slept on it, presumably because it smelled of his owner. The horse settled very quickly with this combination of management, and the jacket became a permanent feature of his routine. I imagine she washed the jacket at some point (!), but wore it first before leaving it with her horse again.

ROLLING AND RUBBING

Rolling (22–25) and rubbing are two more ways in which horses both leave their own scent and take on those of others. Horses can be seen waiting for the chosen rolling patch in a paddock to become free before taking their turn to roll and have a good scratch, a self-massage and to contribute their own personal smell to it as well as taking up the combination herd smell. I find that it is often the lowest-ranking horses who roll first, with the most senior having the last go, presumably to leave their scent as the most obvious one. Some yards, where the horses are not turned out, have a dedicated sand pit, or similar, so that they can at least roll in hand, and they usually do so enthusiastically. In these cases it seems a good plan to note where horses appear to be in the captive herd rank order, and to let them roll in turn in that order. (Many people believe that horses do not have rank orders, but, conversely, many others do. There are also those who recognize that horses do have rank orders, but believe their function is defined by and limited to competition for scarce resources.)

Fences, tree trunks and branches are all convenient rubbing posts for horses. Most owners seem to enjoy watching their horses roll, but try to stop them rubbing in case they not only spoil their manes and tails but rub themselves to excess and become sore. If this is happening, protective clothing can be worn but, as always, it is better to try to discover the cause of the excessive rubbing (e.g. sweet itch or some other allergy, excessive starch in the diet from cereals, mites, lice) and eliminate it. A normal level of rubbing should be encouraged, because it not only gives pleasure to the horse, but is another way of depositing body smells and also of cementing relationships and creating a cohesive herd.

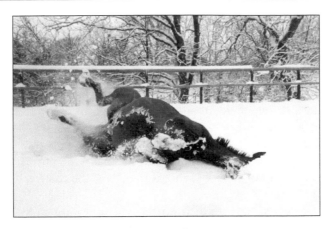

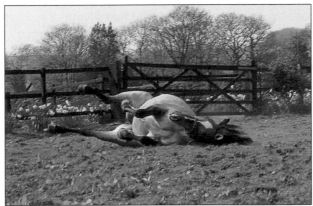

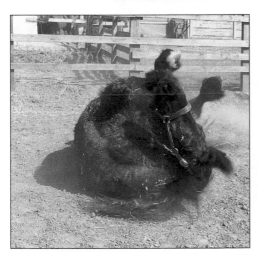

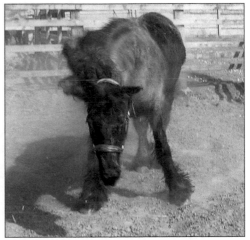

22–25 Rolling is very important and enjoyable to horses. Like most animals, they love rolling and playing in fresh snow (22), on grass (23), and in mud or dust (24). Always watch for a moment when a horse gets up from rolling (25), as rolling can be a sign of abdominal pain. If the horse or pony shakes itself, as here, it almost certainly does not have that problem.

TRACKER HORSES?

For how long can a horse recognize a smell in the air and on objects such as buildings, trees or the ground? Casual reports and incidents from my own experience suggest that on a still day smells can linger for many hours and horses can detect and follow them. Certainly, horses allowed to smell the droppings of other horses on the tracks out hacking or in a strange field are always interested in droppings, even those that are days or even a week old or more (26). If permitted, they will often drop their heads when under saddle in order to investigate and follow the trail of another horse, just like a dog. I have found that they only do this with horses known to them, although I have been told of stallions who, if they have the chance, do it to follow the trail of any mare in season.

Many riders are very strict with their horses when they are under saddle. They not only do not allow grazing, but do not permit their horse to smell droppings or anything else that seems to interest him. I find that plenty of give and take (with due consideration for safety) makes for a better relationship between horse and human and for a more fulfilled, interested and rounded horse. Denying horses the the use of their sense of smell in such circumstances seems rather petty and unnecessary. Horses soon learn when they are permitted to smell their surroundings during exercise and when they are expected to concentrate on something else. I do not find that it creates a precedent, because the horse takes his cue from the handler's demeanour. He uses all his senses to assess when the situation (created by you) is casual and relaxed or one in which work and 'manners' come first, so there should not be a problem.

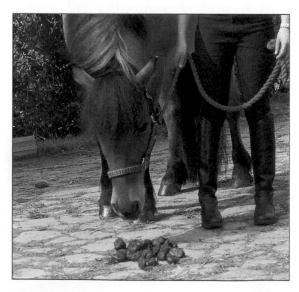

26 Droppings carry important information for horses. By smelling them, they can discover the identity of a horse who has passed that way and when, and its gender and physical and even emotional status. The same applies to urine deposits.

FOOD SELECTION

Horses seem to select their food first by sight and then by smell before risking touching it. Food that to humans has no smell at all clearly has a very different reality for horses. They are impressively skilled at wheedling out objects such as single strands of grass or hay to eat or leave, tiny stones (and the soil as well sometimes) from a clump of turf left in their manger while eating the grass, parts of coarse mixes/sweet feeds they do not like, or medicated pellets. It is fascinating to watch my friend's Fell Pony grazing from the thorniest bushes and taking only the exact leaves she wants, leaving their neighbours on the same stem, without appearing to be pricked by the spikes (27). Horses can graze grass from out of a clump of thistles with no trouble, but I find that they generally avoid stinging nettles unless they are wilted, when they are apparently a good source of vitamin A and other nutrients.

It is a very calming experience watching and listening to a horse swaying and snuffling his way around a field or on the end of a lead as you graze him in hand, his nostrils flaring and closing as he smells out his choices – and they do not all have the same likes and dislikes, either. You can take a horse to water, but you cannot make him drink (if it does not smell right). This is very true and you cannot make him graze where you think fit, either, unless he is the greedy sort. Led horses will take you to their favourite patches, which may look rough and unappetizing, passing by succulent, juicy, young grass on the way. In hand or free, they will raise their heads a little way, sniff the air as if some delightful aroma has titillated their nostrils, then follow their noses to where it came from, if they can possibly reach it.

27 Smell is the first step in the process of choosing food. Even among different ingredients mixed in a bucket, horses can easily sort out what they want to eat and what they do not want to eat. This drawing shows a native pony carefully eating bramble leaves without being pricked by the thorns.

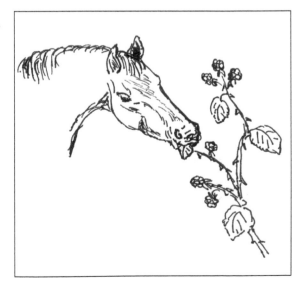

Conscientious owners may wish to pull or cut grass for a horse on box rest, but if you do this, be very sure that it is taken from an area the horse likes, otherwise you will have done an hour or so's back-breaking work filling a tub or net only for your horse to take one sniff and give you a disappointed, disdainful look in rejection of your offering. Foods also clearly smell different at different times of year; whereas a particular bush or patch of grass is avidly sought after in the spring, a few weeks later it is spurned and the horse's attention transferred to something else. Even in winter, horses and ponies will pick and choose their green fodder and by no means eat everything.

We must all have experienced horses who will not eat feed in which they can smell medicine, but, even more exasperating, is the horse who will not eat or even try any or much of the feeds you have so carefully selected and made up for him. These horses may be in a minority, but they are certainly a challenge. When you finally find a type of feed he will eat, you sigh in relief, buy three bags of it and find that, after half a sack, that's it – another one rejected. The problem sometimes seems to be that what smells good to us (e.g. sweet, syrupy, molassed feed with herbs, linseed or mint in it) smells just too much for the horse. Horses in general do not seem to like strong smells (not only strong-smelling feeds, but also alien things such as blood, pigs or strong disinfectants), and although today's practice is usually to buy branded, made-up feeds, whether cubes or coarse mixes, for the difficult feeder something more bland and natural often does the trick; for example, straight grain, if you feed cereals, and chop cut at home from hay or haylage you know your horse will eat. You can always add a broad-spectrum vitamin and mineral supplement if necessary.

There can also be the same problem with hay and haylage. What smells good to us may smell most unappealing to the horse, and although the smell and appearance may be a guide to quality, it is no guide to nutrient content. There is a lot to be said for getting a small sample of hay or haylage for choosy horses to at least give you a guide as to whether or not they are willing to try it. An example of horses acquiring a particular taste is that of hay that smells rather like tobacco. Most horses love this hay but, in fact, it is slightly mowburnt (overheated in the stack) and so not of such good quality and feeding value as hay that has been baled when drier and kept in a better ventilated stack, with spaces left between the bales.

Although, as mentioned above, horses can sort out individual strands of hay or haylage, it can help to introduce them to a new bale from possibly a different farm, field or part of a field (and how is the purchaser to know?) if you start mixing in forage from the new bale before the old one is quite finished. Even the time of day the crop is cut can affect its attractiveness. Hay cut on a warm morning when the sun is climbing high in the sky and the sugars are rising smells much sweeter (that glorious, intoxicating, natural sweetness rather than the contrived sort that comes from a manufacturer's laboratory) than hay from the same field and the same soil cut in the late afternoon or evening when the sun is sinking and the sugar content is falling. Some owners purposely buy second-crop hay or hay that is cut during the night by headlights because it will have little sugar in it and so is safer for their native ponies.

When introducing a new type of feed to a horse, it is best to mix increasing amounts of it with the horse's present feed in order to get him used to the new smell and taste. It has been claimed that plastic containers for feed and water are 'not good' for horses, though the reason for this theory is unclear. Some types of plastic do give off fumes, particularly if wet, which humans cannot detect. However, I did have a problem with one of my mares. I once offered her a feed she turned out not to like from a particular plastic bucket and, despite my having washed it, she refused to eat out of the bucket for several days afterwards, no matter what it contained.

FEEDING TIMES

Although horses do not produce saliva in anticipation of receiving food (they only do so when food, or anything else, is in the mouth), they do show all the usual signs of anticipation when they hear the familiar sounds of their feed being brought round. If the feed room is near the stabling area, they can undoubtedly smell the process, too.

Some highly-strung horses are so stressed by waiting for their feed that they perform stereotypies ('stable vices') while waiting, such as weaving, head twirling, box walking and general pacing around or kicking. It is good management to feed such horses first to reduce their distress, not leave them till last in a futile and misjudged attempt to 'teach them a lesson'. Such an attitude shows a lack of understanding of equine psychology.

In some livery yards it is common to arrange for other owners or yard staff to feed other horses than their own at certain times. The owner will leave the horse's feed ready mixed, although water should not be added until it is given to the horse, as leaving damp feeds standing for some time can make the food very unpalatable. When feeds are left ready for someone else to feed, they should be left not by the stable door, but in the feed room and covered over or left inside the feed bin or a cupboard to reduce the chance of the horses being teased by the smell. Also owners should not leave their horses' breakfasts just outside their boxes every evening for the yard manager to give the next morning; the horses have the mental torment of being able to see and smell their food all night, but not being able to reach it. Even covering it over is not enough to disguise its presence when so close. This alone is bad enough, but if the horses are not left enough forage (hay, haylage or other fibrous feed) to last them through the night and they run out several hours before the morning feed (a very common occurrence), it amounts, in my personal view, to cruelty.

PADDOCK CONTAMINATION

One of the reasons for removing droppings from paddocks is to help limit internal parasite infestation, but droppings left for more than half an hour contaminate the land with their smell. This was discovered more than 30 years ago by Dr Marytavy Archer at the then Equine Research Station in Newmarket, England. Picking up the droppings after this time still left the smell, but spreading the paddocks after the grazing season with cattle manure disguised the equine smell and brought former lavatory areas of the field back into grazing use. Simply resting the land did not have the same effect.

THERE'S WATER AND THERE'S WATER

A horse's most important nutrient is water, and a horse who will not drink is even more worrying than one who will not eat. Depending on temperature, sweat levels and, particularly, humidity, dehydration can set in quickly. A horse left standing sweating in a stuffy stable or vehicle on a hot day, and especially on a humid day, can become significantly dehydrated in a very few hours without doing any work. If he is away from home or in an unfamiliar yard and doesn't like the smell of the water offered to him, this can cause real problems. However, in any weather a free, clean water supply is as vital to horses as to humans, but it has to be water the horse will accept. Just as some horses will go hungry and lose weight rather than eat bad or unappetizing food, so some horses will become dehydrated if offered water they do not fancy. The smell alone can put them off; often they will not even taste it.

There is a wide variety of water supplies, and this includes mains water, rainwater and water from streams, springs, rivers and ponds. Whatever one's views on mains water with its added chemicals, there is no doubt that it is almost always safe for humans and horses to drink, barring the occasional accident. However, troughs in fields fed from mains water can still cause illness if they are not cleaned out regularly. This is because decomposing dead birds or other animals, or algae and other organisms, can get into the trough. Rainwater should normally be safe, but even this may be suspect, depending on the surface it has run over before being directed into gutters and downspouts to be stored in a butt. Rivers and streams may contain chemical pollutants (e.g. fertilizers, herbicides, insecticides and leaks from industrial sources) and ponds are very often stagnant. In my experience, horses do not seem to be able to differentiate between water that is safe and water that is not. If horses are out on a long ride or away at a competition, for example, if the water smells and tastes alright, they will drink it if they want to.

On one occasion, a friend's horse, a particularly sensitive individual, suffered a mystery illness that her vet could only put down to the fact that the small yard's main supply of water came from a stream on their land. He suggested that a rotting carcase further upstream could be the cause of pollution that was causing the horse's illness, although all the other horses and ponies were unaffected.

People who compete regularly may rely on being able to water their horses at the competition venue and find that, at some places, the horses will not drink even mains water. In cases like this it is a good idea to take a large camping container full of drinking water from home. 'Foreign' water may be disguised by adding things to it (e.g. water in which sugar beet pulp has been soaked, provided it has not fermented). An acquaintance always adds a tiny dash of mint cordial to her horses' water at home and away and finds that this nearly always works. Horses used to going on long rides do get used to drinking from whatever source is offered, and competitive endurance horses, for example, are encouraged to drink from any available source *en route*.

The sense of smell also comes into play on the way home. Most horses show signs of recognizing when they are nearing home, even if they cannot see much out of their vehicle. It could be that they recognize the smell of the air as they near home.

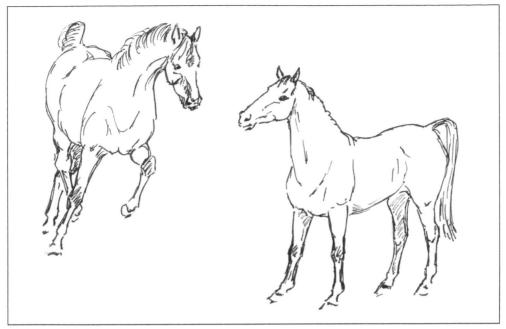

28 Stallions use their acute sense of smell to detect whether or not a mare is in season and the stage of her season. Most mares will voluntarily only accept the stallion towards the end of their season.

BREEDING

Because the breeding instinct in horses is so strong, it is not surprising that stallions can smell a mare in season up to about a mile away if the wind is blowing in the right direction (28). The smell of a mare in oestrus is so compelling that stallions have been known to break or jump out of their paddock and also their stable if the fencing or doors have not been high enough or substantial enough. A few years' ago, there was a photograph in an equestrian magazine of a competition stallion who not infrequently jumped over a two-metre high fence surrounding a small enclosure outside his stable if there was a mare in season within smelling distance.

In domestic conditions, stallions and in-season mares who have not been previosuly introduced normally meet at a trying bar or barrier so that the stallion can test whether or not the mare is ready to be mated. This way the stallion is protected from kicks should the mare not be ready to mate. The stallion and mare should be allowed to sniff nostrils and smell each other's bodies as far as they are able. The stallion will smell and lick the mare around her tail and vulva and, if the mare allows this and gives all the usual signs of being full in season and accepting the stallion's enquiries (e.g. dribbling mucus and urine and 'winking' [opening and closing the vulva]), they are taken elsewhere to a covering yard or area and mated in hand. Mares also often approach stallions themselves.

Stallions who run with their mares should have new mares introduced to them, and their existing herd if any, when they are firmly not in season. In this way, acceptance by the other mares is more likely and the new mare's introduction to the stallion is likely to be fairly uneventful. In natural conditions the stallion is with his mares all the time. Left to arrange their own affairs, which domestic breeding equines are not usually allowed to do, wise stallions will approach a mare from the side (avoiding both sets of hooves and also her teeth) in order to smell her and check whether or not she is in season. The pheromones the mare gives off vary according to the stage of her cycle and stallions are adept at knowing just when a mare is ready to mate – and so are mares. They will then sniff nostrils and the stallion will smell the mare's body and particularly her groin and tail area to check her condition. Usually, with an experienced stallion, there is no problem.

Despite proper introductions, it is not a good idea to expect a first-time stallion or maiden mare to know instinctively exactly what to do. In nature, horses learn not only how to meet other horses, but they also see horses mating and learn this way. In domestic conditions this does not normally happen, so it is wiser to let green stallions mate experienced mares and vice versa.

Stallions either urinate or defecate not only on top of the droppings of their own mares, possibly to indicate 'ownership', but also on top of the droppings of other males in the region to warn them that this area and these mares are their property. Afterwards, they often turn and smell their own deposits, maybe just to make sure that they have done a proper job of masking other smells.

The smell of the urine and mucus that a mare passes when in season stimulates the stallion's libido even more, and horses allowed to court before mating, ideally at liberty but also in hand, are known to have higher conception rates than those not given this time or opportunity. Mares tested by a teaser stallion but mated by another stallion also have lower conception rates.

Once the mare goes out of season the stallion is not stimulated sexually by her smell and she will fend off sexual advances vigorously, but friendship remains in a herd where the stallion lives with his mares.

The various smells of mare and foal are crucial in helping each to recognize the other and to bond. Immediately after foaling the mare will smell and lick her new arrival all over, and this process firmly establishes the foal's smell and taste in the mare's mind. Similarly, the foal remains very close to or touching the mare for several hours or even a few days after foaling and absorbs her smell and taste. In a breeding herd, a mare uses smell more than sight to identify any other foal who might want an illicit drink from her and she may reject it quite harshly.

In cases of bereaved mares or foals, smell is also vital in establishing a successful adoption. Various methods have been recommended to encourage a mare to accept another foal, such as draping it with her dead foal's skin, rubbing it with her afterbirth if this is practical, or smearing its muzzle with some of her own milk. A little of her own dung or urine spread elsewhere on the orphan foal's coat may also provide her with a familiar smell and so encourage acceptance. A further step advocated by some is to smear a little of a strong smelling substance (e.g. an anticongestant ointment or liquid [diluted menthol or eucalyptus aromatherapy oils, or a branded product such as Vick]) just inside the mare's nostrils in order to confuse her detection of the strange foal's scent. The main difficulty is in getting the mare to accept the foal rather than the other way round, but done carefully and sensibly adoption can be successful.

Stallions taking over a feral herd of mares and their offspring have been regularly reported as killing young foals sired by the previous stallion, but not their own foals. A stallion's own foals probably smell something like him, so he can smell which are his and which are his predecessor's. It is thought that this behaviour could be due to an instinct of the stallion to promote his own genes rather than permit the continuation of those of another.

AROMATHERAPY

Aromatherapy is a very popular complementary therapy. It aims to treat physical and emotional problems by allowing the horse (or human or other animal) to inhale the scents (the physical particles given off) of essential plant oils, either 'neat' or blended into a base oil. Aromatherapy was a well-used therapy in ancient times and never really fell out of use. Throughout civilization, scented plants, both dried and fresh, have been hung in homes, scattered on floors, used as massage oils and burned in waxes and oils. For example, the seeds of lavender (a well-known healing plant and very versatile oil) scattered on carpets, trodden in for a day or so, then swept or vacuumed up, not only scent the carpet but repel carpet mites and other insects, clean and condition the fabric, kill bacteria and perfume the room all at the same time. Aromatherapy became a healing art of both body and mind. Healers selected aromas not only to disguise the pungent smells common in people and homes due to what we would today term a lack of hygiene, but also because it was realized that specific aromas had a noticeable beneficial effect on particular conditions.

Because animals have a much more highly developed sense of smell than humans, they are normally very interested in aromas, and horses appear to be particularly susceptible to them. The oils are extracted from plants and are concentrated to become up to a hundred times stronger than the levels normally found in the source plants. They are concentrated chemicals and, as such, most must be blended in bland base oils such as grape seed oil or almond oil. Two that can be applied neat are lavender and tea (or tee) tree. For horses, they are normally offered to the horse to inhale or are massaged gently into his body. Sometimes, they are offered to horses to lick off the hand, and it is interesting to note that they usually do this with the underside of the tongue, as substances seem to be more easily absorbed there. (It is usually recommended that homoeopathic remedies are also placed under the tongue, where possible.)

How Does Aromatherapy Work?

Scents do have an effect on our state of mind and it is now widely accepted that the mind can certainly affect the body. The particles of a scent can pass through the skin and the mucous membranes in the nasal and air passages and so into the blood and lymph. They can be very effective in helping with emotional and stress-related conditions as well as physical ones. Some oils have antibacterial properties and are believed to aid healing by helping to adjust the body's biochemistry.

Conditions for which aromatherapy is used include injuries such as sprains, bruises and wounds; osteoarthritis; stress relief; emotional problems such as trauma, anxiety, depression, fear and sadness; digestive disorders; parasite infestations and other skin conditions; infections; impotence; and internal and external tissue damage.

Selecting and Using the Oils

A trained aromatherapist will discuss the horse's history and current problems with the owner, bearing in mind any veterinary diagnosis, then select whatever oils are felt to be appropriate. However, the main selection is made by the horse himself.

The oils come in small, brown, glass bottles to protect the contents from sunlight. Up to five or six oils can be tried at any one session. The therapist will make a fist with his/her hand and put the bottle inside it with its top level with the top of the fist (29). This is so that there is no glass protruding, which the horse might try to grasp with his teeth and possibly break. The bottle is then offered to the horse to sniff. As with feed selection, horses seem to know what they need; also, certain scents are appealing while the horse is in a particular condition or has a particular problem, perhaps rather like pregnancy cravings. He will use first one nostril then, if at all interested, the other. If he does this, and especially if he continues to sniff the bottle and perhaps tries to lick it, that is the oil he needs. If he turns his head away and is either uninterested or repulsed by the scent, that particular oil is inappropriate at that time.

The therapist will make up a blend of oils in a base oil for the owner either to let the horse inhale or to massage onto his neck or breast (30). If the oil is to be used topically on, for example, a skin disorder, it is massaged gently into the relevant area and may be inhaled as well.

Horses' needs may change from day to day and even at different times of day. It is not possible to keep calling the therapist back, so the usual advice is to offer the single oil or blend as instructed and note when the horse loses interest. At this point, that particular aroma has done its job and, hopefully, helped the horse. Or, perhaps, another selection is needed.

Oils must be kept well away from animals, children and irresponsible people in general; they are medicines after all. Therapists (and owners) should not lend their oils to anyone else, because they are their responsibility and, in their absence, they cannot control what other people may do with them. They should be kept in a cool, dark place, if necessary locked up.

Other Sources of Scents

Fans of vampire films and stories will remember that garlic keeps the vampires away. I cannot speak for vampires, but peeled garlic hung near doors and windows does seem to help repel insects. Dried lavender is also a traditional insect repellent that can be hung up in stables. Crushed garlic rubbed around doors and open window frames does the same job. The old farmers' practice of hanging up cut onions in animal houses plays a similar role and is said with conviction to be very effective at keeping away respiratory diseases and allergies. My experience is that this does work and I have always done it with my horses, though the onions must be changed frequently. A small number of horses make a habit of eating the onions, but most horses leave them alone or have just one attempt at eating them. One attempt is usually a sufficient deterrent!

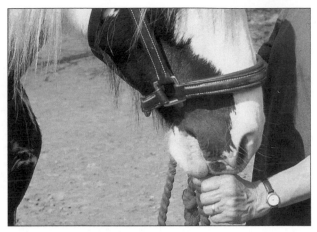

29 Selecting aromatherapy oils. The small bottle should be held inside the fist with the top level with the index finger so that the horse cannot bite and break it. The horse will smell it and quickly decide whether or not it is the one he requires. He may then smell it for several seconds and may try to lick it.

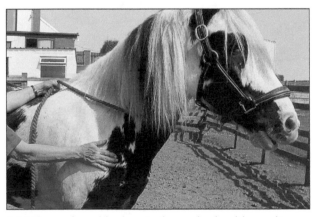

30 Oils can be rubbed on to the neck, shoulder and/or chest, from where the horse can easily inhale their aroma. Here, lavender oil is being used to help calm down a sensitive horse.

Horses have access to a whole sensory world of scents that is almost completely denied to humans. This needs to be borne in mind when faced with unaccountable behaviour and it is important to try to please, and not offend, horses with the smells that are all around them in a domestic environment.

Chapter 9
THE SENSE OF TASTE

The sense of taste is intricately interwoven with that of smell, and much of what has been said about smell applies to taste.

FOOD AND TASTE

Once a horse has smelt his chosen food and decided that it seems appealing, is what he needs at that particular time, is familiar or is recognized as something good, he takes it into his mouth for tasting (**31**). At this point the horse may decide to keep it there, chew it and swallow it or, at any time during this process, he may change his mind and drop it out of his mouth if it does not come up to expectations or is actually repulsive (e.g. most poisonous plants or food that has gone 'bad').

The flavour of food depends on its blend of both smell and taste. As horses can detect only the tastes of salt, sour, bitter and sweet, any other sensation must come from the smell, which contributes to the overall flavour. Whether a food tastes good or mediocre seems to determine digestive efficiency in that it stimulates the production of digestive juices in the gut. Horses, like humans and other animals, note the taste, texture and flavour (smell and taste) of their food; of these, the sense of

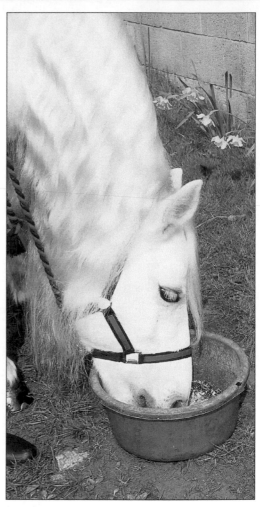

31 After smelling food, a horse will then taste it. He may decide to eat it or he may drop it out of his mouth if he does not like the taste of it.

taste is probably the most important. A horse is what he eats, so a healthy appetite must determine to a large extent whether or not he has a healthy body and, also, mind. 'Mood food' is the current buzz phrase in the horse world as clinical nutrition becomes better understood in relation to equine physiology, behaviour and performance.

The taste of anything in the mouth is best distinguished in a moist environment. The horse's natural food, grass, is almost always moist, unless it has become shrivelled during a drought. In periods of drought, horses have been known to die of impaction colic due to eating dried-up, shrivelled grass, despite having plenty of drinking water available. Moist or wet food is more natural and comfortable for horses to eat, and presumably they can taste it better as well.

At one time the advice was that horses should be fed dry food. This was because it was thought that if water was added to the food, it would dilute the digestive juices and cause poor digestion, despite the fact that grass and herbage, the horse's natural foods, usually contain a lot of water. The horse world is still full of strange concepts and theories and this one is an excellent example of not thinking through an idea. Saliva is intended to further soften up food and make it easier to chew and swallow and, also, to start the digestive process. It is much less acid than the stomach juices. Adding water to the feed can only enhance the job of the saliva, not interfere with digestion. Dry feed is known to be instrumental in causing choke in horses (where dry and imperfectly chewed food clogs in the oesophagus or gullet), so now the advice generally is to feed damp feed, although cubes or pellets are normally fed dry. Coarse mixes/sweet feeds are moist in themselves and should not need dampening, although it would do no harm. Dampened feed should be fed very soon after adding the water, as otherwise it can become mouldy and cause digestive disorder.

POISONING

Poisons are substances that can harm or even kill a horse or interfere with its physiological functioning. Some poisonous substances are used in carefully controlled amounts for treating disorders; if too much is given the horse can be harmed or killed. To be harmful, most poisons need to be absorbed into the blood and transferred around the body to the various tissues they are capable of harming. A crucial task of the liver is to detoxify poisons; however, in the process it too can become damaged and inflamed, a fact that can be discovered by means of a blood test to check liver function.

Toxins can form on 'bad' food that has been damaged by exposure to the weather and has become contaminated by moulds and/or bacteria, or has simply started to rot as part of the normal decomposition process of all organic, dead matter. Some animals acquire a taste for some poisons, and these are taken in by mouth. Poisonous substances can also be administered to horses by injection, by absorption through the skin or by inhalation.

In cases of digestive colic, feed that has not been digested properly can begin to decompose in the gut. Toxins then form and the horse becomes ill. An example of this is when horses are fed too much starchy feed (e.g. cereal grains and grain-containing feeds). If the amount of starchy feed is more than can be processed in the small intestine, the excess is pushed on into the large intestine, which is not equipped to process such food. This is why there is a guideline of not feeding a horse more than 4.4 lb of cereals/concentrates in one feed, as this is about as much as a horse's stomach and gut can cope with at one time.

A good way to feed cereals is to mix them in with generous amounts of chopped fibre (32) so that the horse is taking in more fibre by volume than cereals. This can be achieved by buying branded feeds that contain few cereals in relation to their other ingredients, or by filling a tub or large manger with one of the short-chopped forage feeds currently available and mixing cereals into it. The old horsemen's way of mixing a horse's concentrates (often called 'hard feed') with a good double handful or two of chop (hay, often with some feeding straw such as oat straw, chopped up to about 1.6 in) helped to ensure that the horse had to eat slowly, chewing each mouthful and taking in only a small amount of cereal at each mouthful.

Today, chop is often incorrectly referred to as chaff. Chaff is the outside husk of cereal grains. Chop is the correct and more descriptive term because it is, in fact, chopped hay and straw. Chopped forages with a high proportion of straw in them should be avoided, because a high straw intake is known to favour the occurrence of digestive blockages.

Oats have long been a favoured cereal grain for horses in hard work, not least because their outside husk is included in the feed with the grain. In my experience barley can be an excellent grain, but it has very little husk, and maize or corn has none at all. Anyone still in the habit of using 'straight' grains (grains/cereals alone without the addition of other ingredients) could, with advantage to their horses, consider adopting the practice of adding a good helping of chop to each feed.

Horses usually love cereals, which tend to taste fairly sweet, and they often bolt them down without thoroughly chewing them. This does not help digestion. In any case, proper dental checks and, if necessary, treatment should be carried out at least once a year for mature horses and more often for young and old ones.

Another example of food decomposing in the gut is when there is a blockage in the large intestine (often at the narrow pelvic flexure and usually when coarse, woody

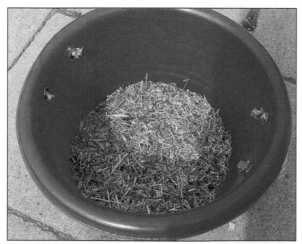

32 Short-chopped forage/fibre feed. This type of feed is normally made from chopped hay, straw, dried grasses and legumes such as alfalfa (lucerne) or, more rarely, vetches or clover. These feeds can be used as hay or haylage replacers in times of scarcity and they are available with different nutrient levels and content, according to a horse or pony's needs.

fibre with a high lignin content is fed, such as large amounts of straw). The blockage causes what horsemen call impaction colic; the food cannot pass onwards and eventually begins to decompose in the gut. The toxins and gases that then form cause great pain in the abdomen.

Symptoms of Poisoning

Some signs of poisoning present themselves quite quickly, but others only start to show when the horse or pony has been slowly poisoned over a period of time. Signs include dullness, jaundice (yellow tinge to mucous membranes), diarrhoea, constipation, loss of gut sounds/movements, excessive gut sounds, colic/abdominal pain, laminitis, blood in the urine, sensitivity to external stimuli such as noise, light and touch, loss of consciousness, abnormal pulse rate, abnormal temperature, convulsions, drooling, incoordination, dilation or constriction of the pupils and distressed breathing. If a horse shows any of these symptoms, veterinary assistance should be sought immediately.

Poisonous Plants

Horses dislike bitter tastes and, it seems, many poisonous plants taste bitter when alive and growing, losing their bitterness when dead and wilted either in the paddock or in conserved forage such as hay, haylage or straw. Although horses do seem to have a sense of what Dr Marthe Kiley-Worthington has described as 'nutritional intuition' in relation to selecting what they need, some horses do eat poisonous plants, but normally only when other more inviting food sources are scarce or absent. Occasionally, though, horses develop a taste for a particular poisonous plant in the same way that humans acquire a taste for unpleasant tasting foods or substances, and they will eat it even when there is plenty of palatable grass around. Therefore, it is always worth checking grazing paddocks regularly and taking appropriate steps to eradicate any poisonous plants found (see Table 1). Sometimes, these are trees and shrubs, which are not so easy to get rid of, but they can be fenced around so that the horses cannot reach them.

Table 1: Some poisonous plants (UK and USA).

UK		USA	
Beech	Holly (berries)	Bracken fern	Red maple
Box	Horse chestnut	Castor bean	Russian knapweed
Bracken	Ivy	Fiddleneck	Tansy ragwort
Buttercup	Laburnum	Golden weed	Whitehead
Daffodil	Oak	Horsetails	Wild cherry
Deadly nightshade	Privet	Jimsonweed	Wild onion
Foxglove	Ragwort	Locoweed	Wild tobacco
Hemlock	Thorn apple	Oleander	Woody aster
Hogweed	Yew	Prince's plume	Yellow star thistle
		Rattleweed	Yew

It is important to ensure that the fencing will keep out large and small horses and ponies. Ponies are often expert 'limbo' artistes and they can get under fencing in ways that you would not have believed possible had you not seen it for yourself, and this includes electrified fencing (33, 34).

If you are in the position of finding poisonous plants in your horse's paddock and the land is owned by an uncooperative landowner who will not take steps to remove them, you can help to safeguard your horse until you find somewhere safer for him to graze by making sure that he is not hungry when turned out. Turning a horse out on a 'full stomach' helps to stop him experimenting with poisonous plants that are normally, but not always, eaten only when the horse is trying something less appealing because he is hungry (35, 36). One pony taken in by an equine charity ultimately died because, out of hunger, he had been chewing old lead-containing roofing felt on a chicken cabin in his field. Another suffered poisoning due to chewing creosote-treated wooden rails in his, to him, bare paddock.

Providing another forage source in the paddock may also help to dissuade horses from feeling obliged to try poisonous plants; they will not feel so hungry. Hay, haylage or large tubs of short-chopped forage would fill the bill. Whatever is provided, it has to be something horses like and will, therefore, eat. Giving short feeds (concentrates) is not so effective, as horses fairly soon feel hungry again after eating them, whereas with ample forage feeds they can eat for many hours.

Insecticides, herbicides and fertilizers can be poisonous to horses and, if these are used on land grazed by horses, it is strongly advised that the label on the container is checked and the length of time noted that must elapse before it is safe for horses to be returned to the land. With some products it is necessary to avoid the land for weeks, whereas other products are safe as soon as they are dry. Horses cannot be relied on to avoid poisonous substances, even artificial ones.

Although the horse's taste buds occur mainly on the tongue, the palate and the back of the throat (the pharynx), a small experiment was carried out on a Welsh cob that suggested that there is also some kind of taste bud or buds in the lips. As a livery client, the owner had no control over the management of the fields where the horses grazed. The finding of ragwort (*Senecio jacobea*) was not uncommon, but to date there had been no cases of ragwort poisoning. The owner offered the cob a tiny piece of ragwort to see if he would eat it. He took a piece of growing leaf and offered it to the cob, who sniffed it, decided to try it, opened his lips and held it, but then dropped it quickly. At no time did the cob's teeth part and his tongue certainly did not touch the ragwort (he was observed very closely), but he still detected a bitter taste after deciding from its smell that the ragwort was worth testing further and picking it up with his lips.

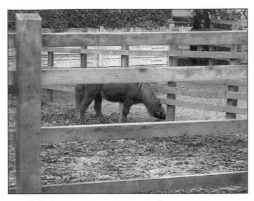

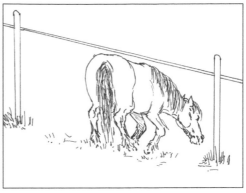

33 This pony is prone to laminitis so has his grazing rationed. When not on grass, he cranes his neck under the fence of his enclosure (where there is hay for him and his companion) and often gets down on his knees and maybe drops onto his shoulder to reach further into the grass paddock.

34 The pony in 33 even 'limbos' under the electric fence to get to grass, although he has never been caught on camera because he does not do it if he knows anyone is watching.

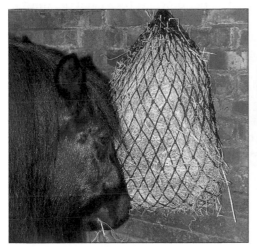

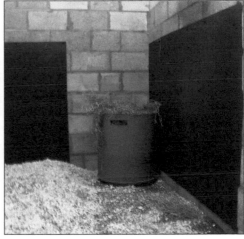

35 Horses are much less likely to sample poisonous plants if they are not hungry when turned out. A generous, but appropriate, ration of tasty hay or haylage is not only filling and nutritious, but it also has great entertainment value. Haynets, used here for a pony, should be tied at head height so that they are reasonably comfortable to eat from. If the haynet sags too low as it empties, the horse can get a hoof or shoe caught if he paws at it.

36 Long forage can be given in containers such as this large tub, which can be fastened to the wall if the horse is likely to move it. Permanently fixed hay containers are available as well. These holders let horses eat naturally with their heads down, which is more comfortable, probably enhances the digestive process and more natural dental wear as the lower jaw drops forward slightly in this position, and encourages relaxation and stretching of the horse's neck and back. It also aids drainage of airways.

Removing Poisonous Plants

Large trees and poisonous shrubs can be chopped down or dug up, but if for any reason this is not an option, they should be securely fenced off for several metres around them so that horses (and ponies and foals) cannot reach them.

Other plants may need spraying if present in large numbers. Small numbers can be dug or pulled up, but you need to be sure that you remove every tiny bit of root (extremely difficult), as some plants, particularly ragwort, spread from the smallest piece left in the soil. Hand pulling is often recommended for ridding land of ragwort, but this can simply make matters worse. A special tool is occasionally advertised, which is claimed to make uprooting ragwort more reliable.

In the UK, good up-to-date advice can be obtained from the Equine Services Department of The Department for the Environment, Farming and Rural Affairs (DEFRA – phone number in the local directory). In the USA, the local County Extension Agent should be contacted. Plants are not all susceptible to the same chemicals, so a product specifically made for one plant may not kill another. It is important to check the label or instruction leaflet to see what the product will kill and also for how long the land will be out of use as regards grazing. A general herbicide should not be bought, as this will kill the grass and any herbs as well. Advice should be taken from a suitably qualified expert. Some plants spread only by seeding, so removing them before they go to seed is effective, but others spread from the roots as well all through the growing season.

Poisonous plants, whether dug up, hand pulled or sprayed, must be taken right out of the paddock and burned or disposed of according to any local bye-laws. Leaving any at all in the paddock where horses can get at them may result in poisoning, as the plants often lose their bitter taste when wilted and dead. This can be a problem if they are present in hay or haylage. A useful tip for removing any poisonous plant present in small numbers is to cut off the plant at ground level, put a handful of salt on the remaining stump, water it in, then add a little more salt. This certainly removed the ragwort from a friend's lawn, so is well worth a try.

FEEDS AND FEEDING

A horse's taste for particular foods develops early in life and it can be quite difficult to persuade some horses to accept what are to them strange tasting foods later in life (37). Horses raised on conventional bloodstock pasture (mainly ryegrasses with some timothy, some clover, but little else – the famous 'green desert' pasture) often will not graze other grasses in a more naturally mixed pasture consisting of herbs and a wide range of grasses, which would provide a more natural diet. (It has been calculated that natural, wild pasture contains well over 100 different types of grasses, herbs and other plants and a figure of 150 types has been quoted.)

I have always been used to grazing my horses out in hand in addition to their normal time turned out, and find it interesting to note which grasses and other plants they like or do not like – and their choices are sometimes perplexing. The horse who had the most restricted tastes would only graze on ryegrass and white clover. I would purposely take her to patches of various other juicy-looking plants that I felt were good for her; for example, herbs (she would not even eat dandelions), which she disdainfully

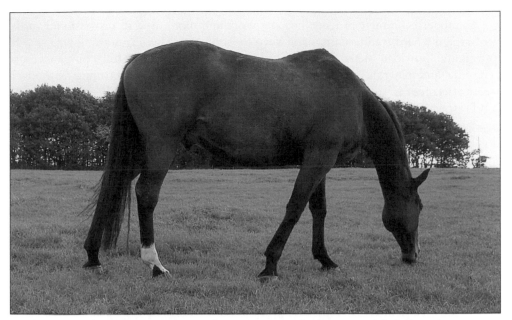

37 There is no doubt that most horses' favourite taste is fresh grass and their favourite situation is head down grazing the grass, an activity horses have evolved to carry out for about two-thirds of their time.

sniffed at before dragging me back to where she wanted to be. This experience confirms the view that traditionally reared Thoroughbreds, as opposed to horses reared on more varied pastures, do go mainly for ryegrasses and white clover because they acquired those tastes on their home studs (USA: stud farms). Such horses, particularly older ones who have been raced, prefer plain, straight rolled oats as their concentrate of choice, presumably because this is what they were brought up to eat, although most will deign to eat others such as branded coarse mixes and cubes.

Some horses may also not eat meadow or mixture hay or haylage for the same reason. So-called racehorse hay is mainly ryegrasses (perennial ryegrass and Italian ryegrass) and extremely limited. Clover hay is almost impossible to get nowadays, as is lucerne (alfalfa) hay. Lucerne hay is sometimes available in its long form, but it is more usually used chopped for branded short-chopped forages, of which it may form all or part of the formulation. Some horses seem to find lucerne hay rather strong (described by one nutritionist as 'rather like strong tea without sugar') and may not eat it unless something sweet is added. A little syrup, molasses or honey, or being mixed with soaked sugar beet pulp, often does the trick. It is a case of finding out what your horse likes.

As modern commercial feeds become more and more used in professional yards, only the die-hard traditionalists still keep to 'straights'. There is nothing wrong with 'straights' provided steps are taken to ensure that a horse's full complement of vitamins and minerals is included in his diet. Because of modern farming methods, it seems that feed is not what it used to be, but equine nutrition has been a recognized and respected science for many years and many modern feeds are excellent. The same goes for ideas on grazing pasture for horses. Increasingly, it is recognized that horses evolved to thrive on a wide variety of herbage, and grass mixes are available that offer good variety and nutrition for horses and ponies in all categories, from potential Derby winners to children's hacks.

Horses raised on a varied diet on the stud and in both stable and field should be less difficult to feed than some of their predecessors. The taste for a wider selection of feedstuffs was acquired early in life.

The food a mare eats affects the taste of her milk and so even before a foal eats solid food he will be exposed to certain tastes from this source. In the same way, milk tastes different at different times of year depending on what the cows are eating (e.g. kale in the autumn, turnips or fodder beet in winter, spring grass at turn-out time, clover in summer). Cows might also graze protein-rich lucerne for a short time in the summer and the milk is noticeably more bitter then, bearing out the belief that 'neat' lucerne is rather unpalatable to some horses.

It is a good plan to give weanlings the concentrates that they have been used to eating when with their dams to help avoid the familiar setback they suffer (from stress) at this time. Therefore, if a horse is being bought as a weanling, information should be given to the new owner on what types of feeds and what brands the youngster is used to. If you are the buyer, you should ask the seller what the young horse has been fed on. Different vitamin and mineral supplements can vary in taste, not to mention hay and haylage. Every effort should be made to have a few weeks' supply of the young horse's hay or haylage sent with him so that the changeover to his new home can be made gradually. This will help the young animal over this major change in his life.

Being bought as a weanling is a double blow for a youngster – he has recently not only lost his dam, but also his familiar companions, human handlers and surroundings. It has been reported that one five-months-old potential performance horse had been weaned on the day of the sale at which he fetched a record price, and he was exhibited jumping! Can anyone truly believe that this is acceptable on the grounds of equine welfare? Many behaviourists and other professionals feel that weaning earlier than is natural leaves permanent psychological scars on many animals. This can lead to behavioural problems throughout life and may well be one reason for horses becoming 'poor doers', highly strung and nervous and/or being difficult to keep in good physical condition and fitness.

Unless there is a very good reason to wean, such as mare and foal not getting on (lack of mare's milk is not a reason, as the foal can be given supplementary feed), foals can be left with their dams until a couple of months before the next year's foal is due. By this time the foal will be taking insignificant amounts of milk from what little the mare is still producing, and both foal and mare will be able to enjoy each other's company, as in nature, and not be put through the considerable stress of enforced, unnaturally early separation and its resultant deleterious effects on both. Commercial interests, such as the dates of weanling sales, can be changed in the interests of equine welfare, if the will is there. In my experience, horses weaned very early for whatever reason often seem to remain mentally immature well into adulthood, showing such 'baby' signs as chewing anything within reach, the inability to concentrate for more than a few minutes, a tendency to shying/spooking at familiar objects, moodiness and erratic behaviour.

Getting a horse used gradually to the taste of a new feed or (particularly) forage is not only wise from a digestive health viewpoint but also from a practical one, as gradually introduced tastes are more likely to be accepted. Mixing a little of the new feed in with the old in gradually increasing amounts is the standard way of doing this. Although many people do this with concentrates, few do so with forages, either short-chopped branded ones or hay or haylage. It is very important to give the microorganisms in the large intestine time to build up adequate populations of the types needed to cope with the new feed so that effective digestion can take place. Otherwise, painful and potentially fatal colic can so easily result from both imperfectly digested fibre and a disrupted complement of microorganisms. A little of the new batch of fibre should always be mixed in with the existing batch in increasing amounts over about two weeks, until the changeover is complete and the older feed is used up.

Many owners are interested in how best to feed their horses. Trouble is taken to find out which of the many advertised brands will, in theory, be most suitable for their particular horses, and those are then bought. How dispiriting it is, then, to find that the horse checks the feed by smell and might, even at that point, baulk. Maybe he will take a mouthful or two, or even eat the feed for a day or two, but then refuse it. Watching for any sign of enthusiasm in a fussy feeder can be an anxious time as he, or more often she, pushes the food around, picking out the tastiest bits and leaving the rest and then standing demanding something more palatable. You can take a horse to water, but you cannot make him drink; and you cannot make him eat, either.

Some horses will eat a feed happily for a few days or weeks and then will stop eating it. With these, rather than adding various goodies to tempt the horse, it is simpler to find two or three types of feed suitable for the horse's needs and to make a constant, very gradual change between them. Sometimes, any range from a particular brand will be refused, but equally you may hit on one or more particular feeds that the horse loves and will eat readily, lessening your stress levels considerably!

Horses, being trickle feeders, naturally evolved to eat for most of their waking hours and they can be expected to eat at most times of day and night if they are healthy. Refusing feed the horse likes, especially if he also refuses a second type he likes, should raise your suspicions that something is wrong. Horses being 'off their feed' is one of the commonest signs of illness, not only of digestive problems, so it is important to look for other symptoms as well, not least excessive fatigue in horses working hard or harder than their fitness levels justify. Learning the basic vital signs for all horses and particularly your own (i.e. temperature, pulse and respiration, behaviour and demeanour, state of hydration [dehydrated horses often will not eat no matter what you offer them], condition of urine and droppings) can give you and your vet useful information as to what might be the problem.

The only time it is normal for equines to eat droppings is when they are foals, who do it to acquire gut microorganisms from their dams' droppings. In adult horses, eating droppings or other non-food substances such as wood, bark or significant amounts of soil is a sign of a depraved appetite, usually because something vital is missing from the diet. This could be adequate fibre to create digestive comfort or specific nutrients, or because the amount of feed is insufficient. It can also happen because of a physiological or metabolic disorder or boredom and during or after a course of antibiotics. The old, and still relevant, treatment was to put some dung from a healthy horse from the same stable in some water and administer it by stomach tube, but today it would be more likely that the horse would be fed prebiotics and probiotics.

Horses who develop a taste for soil may not be short of nutrients. It is not at all unknown for horses in a particular paddock or field to have a favourite spot for licking the earth despite being on perfectly good diets, although if this took up a significant amount of their time I would suggest that their diets were reassessed.

Medicines

Many medicines for horses are presented in paste form to be squirted into the back of the mouth, but some have to be fed in other ways, usually by being put in the feed. Some horses will take them readily, but many will not and owners come up with all sorts of ruses to get the medicine down. Sometimes, a little more than usual of something sweet does the trick (e.g. molasses, honey or soaked sugar beet pulp, or mixing that almost universal favourite of horses into the feed, carrots, grated up fairly finely so that the whole feed is flavoured with it). Mint products of various kinds also often induce a horse to eat a doctored feed, and melted chocolate or toothpaste spread on bread can also be used to disguise the taste of medicine. However, as some mints contain menthol and all chocolate contains caffeine, these will not be appropriate for horses that compete under rules, as they are both prohibited substances, although large amounts would be needed to stimulate and affect the performance.

If your horse is on standard phenylbutazone, which has a rather bitter taste, and you find it difficult to get him to eat his feed with the 'bute' in it, the sachets can be kept in a freezer or a cold refrigerator, as the low temperature reduces the bitter taste. Newer forms of phenylbutazone do not taste so bitter and also do not appear to have the same risk of other unwanted side-effects.

Gentle Persuasion

It is well known that feeding a horse his favourite titbit while he is having some unpleasant task performed on him can get him to associate the task with the pleasant taste of a treat, making the job easier in future, provided you always produce the treat.

Water

Drinking muddy water is often taken to mean that a horse or other animal is short of minerals, but it could simply mean that he does not like the taste of the water that comes out of the yard taps or pipes. This can apply particularly to new horses in a yard, who may take some time to accustom themselves to the possibly different taste of the water in their new home. If a horse consistently drinks muddy water as opposed to apparently clean water, this should certainly be looked into; the different waters should be sampled and an assessment made on the basis of the results. There is also a risk of sand colic in such horses.

If your premises have a pond, stream or other natural source such as a well or a reservoir of rainwater, it is sensible to have it checked for purity fairly often. Ponds are notorious for becoming stagnant or 'thick', especially in dry periods, and all natural sources can become polluted, despite local regulations, from chemicals used on surrounding land or from dead animals and birds rotting in the water. Carcases can be a source of disease in horses. Sadly, horses often seem unable to detect by taste whether or not water is actually safe to drink as opposed to simply acceptable to them.

Horses having access to several choices of water source may choose a favourite, sometimes to the exclusion of the others. This can can cause inconvenience if this source cannot be piped to their stabling for them to drink when they are stabled. Often their favourite water has to be gathered in containers and transported to the stable so that it can be used there, or at least mixed with the piped source. Thankfully, this is fairly rare.

Getting horses to drink water when they are away at competitions or other events can sometimes prove problematic, as mentioned earlier. It can also be a problem if the owner wants to give an electrolyte product after hard and sweaty work, when mineral salts are lost in the sweat. To get their horses used to drinking any water anywhere, some owners or managers habitually put a drop or two of peppermint, apple or cinnamon essence into the horses' drinking water to provide a familiar taste. Many horses also like the taste of the water in which their sugar beet pulp has been soaked, and some of this can be tried in their water to see if it will tempt them to drink. If the competition or outing simply involves a single day away and the horse is known to refuse strange water, you can always take a large container or two of his usual drinking water for him, using the local supply for washing him down, if necessary.

It is a common practice for water buckets to be topped up for quickness rather than regularly changed. Many horses make it very clear by not drinking such water that they think this is a dirty habit, and I agree. Water standing in stables can quickly become tainted by dust and stable debris, horse or bird droppings, the horse's own saliva and part-eaten food and, if the ventilation and bedding management are inadequate, by ammonia in the airspace, which settles on the water and may be absorbed into it. Owners who leave large tubs of water for their horses overnight or when they are at work all day are often tempted to top them up rather than drag them out and empty them at least once a day, scrub them out to remove the dirt and slime that has accumulated, rinse them thoroughly and refill them with clean water. This is just basic hygiene management.

Horses will certainly often go thirsty rather than drink stale, tainted water that has been standing in the stable for some hours. This causes many owners to think that the horse has enough water and is not thirsty, so they fail to change it (one job less to do), either leaving it if there seems to be quite a lot or simply topping it up. The horse becomes thirstier and thirstier and may even become dehydrated. Two checks can be made to discover whether or not a horse is dehydrated. The skin pinch test (38) will expose significant dehydration and the capillary refill test (39) will reveal when a horse is only slightly dehydrated:

- **The skin pinch test.** Pinch up a fold of skin just in front of the horse's shoulder, then let it go again. It should fall flat immediately if the horse is well hydrated, although some experts say that a second's delay is acceptable.
- **The capillary refill test.** For this test, press hard enough with your thumb to leave a white patch on the horse's gum (usually just above one of his corner incisors or front teeth). The area should refill with blood and become pink again within two seconds at most, and preferably sooner for the horse to be adequately hydrated.

Other signs of dehydration are a lack of appetite (and, sometimes, thirst), a dull appearance, lethargy, sunken eyes and, in longer-standing cases, weight loss, smaller amounts of faeces (which are drier than usual), a marked decrease in urination, a weak pulse, acid blood, weakness, depression and, possibly, collapse and unconsciousness.

Watering the Performance Horse

Some years ago it was standard practice to remove not only the feed of a horse due to work strenuously but also his water. Nowadays this is not advised. Water can be left with the horse up to half an hour before his work starts. It passes fairly quickly out of the stomach and on down to the large intestine, which acts as a reservoir in appropriate circumstances. Endurance horses, in particular, are trained to drink en route to prevent or delay the onset of dehydration and fatigue.

After work, the horse can be allowed about three or four swallows every five or ten minutes until he has cooled down and his pulse and respiration have returned to the pre-work warm-up rate. From then on, water can be left with him *ad libitum*.

To persuade a very tired and dehydrated horse to drink, small amounts can be syringed into his mouth with an ordinary plastic syringe so that he gets the taste for the water and may start to drink for himself. The water in which sugar beet pulp has been soaked is sweet and contains some minerals, so is often welcomed by horses after work, including dehydrated ones. Black treacle or molasses dissolved in hot water and added to cold water can be tried as well. In some cases it is necessary for a vet to administer water via a stomach tube.

Materials for Containers

Because they had no taste at all, the old ceramic or glazed earthenware mangers and troughs were excellent if kept clean, and some are still in use. However, if they are cracked or chipped, as most old ones will be, they can harbour infectious agents such as bacteria or viruses, which are harder to eliminate from rough surfaces; however, in practice this is not usually a problem. Ceramic or glazed earthenware mangers are not

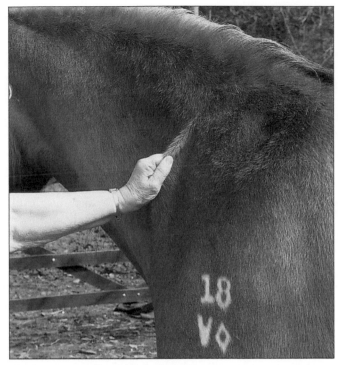

38 Carrying out the skin-pinch test.

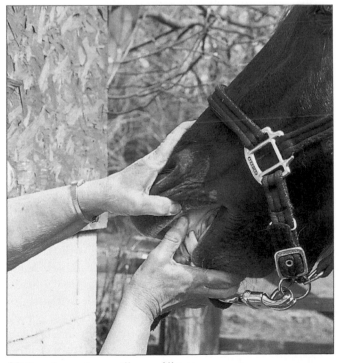

39 Carrying out a capillary refill test.

so convenient to clean as removable ones made of other materials, but this can still be done by using a brush in a bucket of hot soapy water followed by a cloth and cold water for rinsing and removing the soap. There is no need to put in lots of water; it is tricky to get out.

Stainless-steel containers are excellent (if rather expensive), as are enamelled metal ones. Neither of these materials holds tastes or smells if kept clean. Old wooden containers are not hygienic, as wood is absorbent and difficult to keep germ free. Nowadays, plastic or rubber containers of various sorts are mainly used and many of these do certainly hold tastes and have tastes and smells of their own. Some horses will not eat from certain ones, and this can only be discovered by trial and error. Some plastics give off chemicals that taint the feed and water in the containers and this may be why some horses dislike them. They can also cause digestive problems. In practice this does seem rare, although horses should be watched when using plastic or rubber containers to check that they are not being put off (as will some sensitive individuals) and that they are eating and drinking freely.

Although it has nothing to do with taste, it is as well to remember that horses should eat and drink from a low level for ease of ingestion. Having water and feed containers too high can make it uncomfortable for a horse to drink and eat because the gullet/oesophagus is kinked in the throat area. This can result in horses not drinking enough and having difficulty in swallowing. Tubs or buckets on the floor are a cheap and practical way of providing food and water, and they can be stood inside old tyres or fixed to the wall in various ways if the horse is not a quiet feeder or knocks buckets over. Hay containers that allow the horse to eat with his head lower than his withers are readily available or can be made.

Taste in Communication

Because smell and taste are so closely linked, the remarks made above about horses smelling each other or other animals and humans for identification also apply to taste. Horses may lick each other or their familiar and trusted attendants out of friendship, during mutual grooming, to confirm relationship bonds and each other's identity, possibly to acquire salt from sweat and, in the case of mares and foals, to be especially sure of each other's identity so that foals do not risk serious injury from mares not their dams if they approach for milk or protection; mares do not risk wasting their milk on foals not their own.

Orphaned foals, despite being desperately in need of milk, may not take easily to the taste of a foster dam's milk if already used to that of their own dam. Milking the foster dam and carefully and slowly syringing a very little milk at a time into the side of the foal's mouth can help the foal get used to the taste. If the foal has been on a milk substitute after the death of his dam, this can be mixed with the foster dam's milk in gradually decreasing amounts until the foal will suckle readily from her.

From the viewpoint of the dam who has lost her own foal, she can be persuaded to accept an orphan foal either by rubbing its muzzle with her own milk or by rubbing around its tail with her own droppings. Sometimes, her own dead foal is skinned and the skin placed on the orphan, so that she can smell and taste her own foal. In this way, adoption is very often successful. If this is not done, her own afterbirth, if available, can be used instead.

BITS AND TASTE

Unlike dogs and humans, and some other animals, horses' salivary glands are not excited into action by the anticipation or even smell of food, but only by its presence in the mouth. Anything in the mouth stimulates the flow of saliva, even tasteless materials such as stainless steel. Some bits are covered in or made from soft rubber or vulcanite, which is rubber treated at high temperatures with sulphur to harden it and increase its strength. It is generally considered that rubber and vulcanite bits are softer and warmer than metal ones and, therefore, are kinder, but rubber can taste pretty unpleasant.

There are many types of bit made of metal and other materials on the market that have a taste impregnated into them; for example, apple or cinnamon in synthetic bits, or one which is natural to the metal they are made of such as 'sweet iron', copper and certain alloys. These bits are marketed as encouraging the flow of saliva and so helping to keep the mouth soft and responsive. Horse owners read adverts (with persuasive arguments about the taste being inviting to the horse) for these bits and then buy and use them without actually asking someone with a sound background in equine science whether this argument actually holds water, or asking themselves if the horse really looks happy with the situation. Let us pursue this a little in the cause of good riding and equine welfare.

As mentioned above, anything in a horse's mouth, regardless of whether or not it has a specific taste, will encourage the flow of saliva. A flavoured bit may turn on the saliva even more, but some materials actually create a mild irritation of the mouth, which must be unpleasant in itself and similarly appears to kick off the flow of saliva in response.

In riding, even today when many of its finer points have been lost down the genera-tions, people still have a general idea that a horse's mouth needs to be 'wet'. In fact, we should be aiming for the horse to have a moist mouth, because a comparatively 'dry' mouth is believed to hamper the feel, movement and comfort of the bit. Unfortunately, people usually have the mistaken impression that lots of froth in and around a horse's mouth, even slopping on to the ground or splashing on to his chest, shoulders and forelegs, means that he is 'happily mouthing his bit, producing lots of saliva (the more the better) and keeping his mouth soft and receptive', or a theory to that effect.

This is not the case. Excessive salivation in mammals (drooling or frothing) is a sign of distress and dislike. A 'dry' mouth is one of the symptoms of fear. This is because the body is preparing for flight or fight and the sympathetic nervous system is preparing the body for energy use, as in galloping, as opposed to energy acquisition or storing, as in eating, so even the comparatively small amount of saliva needed to keep the tissues of the mouth comfortably moist decreases.

Most horses showing copious (excessive) amounts of froth and, which follows, could be considered as distressed are:

• Ridden with an unrelenting, firm or even hard bit contact, either rigid or varying.
• Ridden or trained by riders with poor hands and/or using harsh techniques.
• Prone to grinding their teeth (a sure sign of anxiety and distress).
• Prone to excessive champing of the bit (if the noseband is loose enough) rather than gentle mouthing.

- Tacked up with bits too high, giving them a constant stop/slow down signal on the corners of the lips, particularly when combined with a significant contact via the reins; if the rider's legs are simultaneously telling them to go, horses find these conflicting aids most confusing.
- Tacked up with nosebands so tight that they cause severe discomfort and even pain, and the horse cannot 'mouth the bit' never mind 'give' to it.
- Forced to tolerate a bit that tastes awful to them or feels uncomfortable or is potentially or actually painful.
- Required to work with a head and neck posture that brings the front line of the face behind (sometimes well behind) or even just approaching the vertical. This deprives the horse of forward vision because of the way his eyes work (he can only see downwards with his head in this position).
- Suffering from neglected teeth and mouth.

An argument against using bits at all has been put forward by Professor Robert Cook, an Englishman who has lived and worked in America for many years. He has designed a bitless bridle, the use of which he considers more humane than riding with a bit. His argument is that a bit triggers the production of saliva and many riders require their horses to go with a head position flexed at the poll ('on the bit' or even behind the vertical), which makes it difficult or impossible for the horse to swallow because of the 'kinking' and, therefore, obstruction of the oesophagus at the throat in this posture (40). The horse feels the need to swallow the saliva, but cannot do so. From discussion with others, it seems that some of this saliva may well also get into the nasal passages and run down out of the nostrils, the horse's only route of air intake and expulsion. He must clearly find all this uncomfortable. Obviously, a good deal of this saliva will contribute to the drooling and frothing seen by many horses ridden in this way.

Some people cover bits with various materials with the aim of making the bit feel soft and squashy and, so it is felt, more comfortable. While the theory is fine, careful thought should be given to what mateial is going to be used to cover the bit. Chamois leather is a common choice, but leather certainly tastes awful to humans (no guide perhaps, as some horses regularly chew leather). One owner used to cover all her horses' bits with Adhesive bandages (sticking plasters) adhesive tape and claimed that, when soaked in saliva, the horses loved them. However, as Adhesive bandages (sticking plasters), even without its medicated pad section, smells 'medical' and presumably tastes the same, this may not be a fully thought out choice.

How else can we tell whether or not a horse is happy with the bit chosen for him? As far as taste is concerned, one should look closely at the horse's face for any sign of tightened skin, tension, moving the bit a lot or trying to do so, a troubled or cross look in the eye, ears back a bit, shaking the head or the horse actually trying to get the bit out of his mouth and drooling. One of my mares, when fitted with a rubber pelham, stood with her head vertical to the ground, her mouth wide open and shook her head from front to back and side to side to try to dislodge the bit. Needless to say, it was removed promptly. A stainless steel one turned out to be ideal for her.

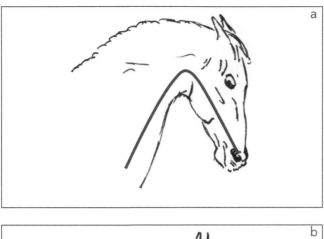

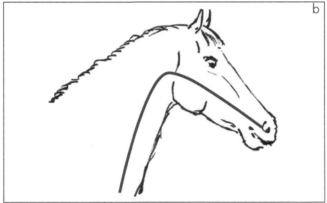

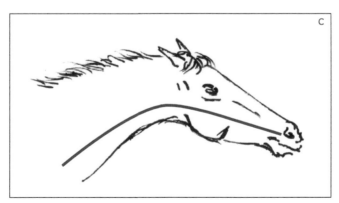

40 Diagrammatic representation of how the structures in a horse's throat area are affected by his head carriage. The first diagram (a) shows the compression, here in the posture, commonly induced in much 'school' riding and mistakenly understood to be, and called, 'on the bit'. Not only can the horse not see far ahead (see p. 103), but he cannot breathe freely or swallow his own saliva. The second diagram (b) shows a normal head carriage, with a free throat area. The third diagram (c) shows the straighter line of the windpipe of a horse in gallop, which permits maximum air flow.

It is reasonable to suppose that a pleasant taste in the horse's mouth should create pleasant associations with the bit and, all else being equal, with being ridden. The best answer to all this (given a correct fit as detailed in the chapter on the Sense of Touch, p.134) is to use a comfortable bit that tastes of nothing at all; stainless steel and the metal brand named Kangaroo come into this category. There must be no inserts such as rollers or 'lozenges' of other tasted metal. The horse should be offered his favourite treat immediately before putting his bridle on. This will get his jaws moving and some saliva flowing. Another piece of the treat could be given after the bridle and noseband have been fastened and checked for comfort. This will leave a nice taste in the horse's mouth and a good impression of the whole procedure for possibly the whole session.

HERBALISM

Herbalism seems to be a particularly suitable therapy for horses, as horses are herbivores and herbs are plants. Hippocrates said 'let food be your medicine and medicine be your food' and this applies to animals every bit as much as humans. Herbalism is surely the oldest therapy in the world and it is frightening, today, that so many plants are being brought to extinction by our actions before we even know what good they can do for us and our animals. Humans were certainly already skilled at using plants as medicine when the earliest written and artistic records were being made thousands of years ago. Domestic dogs treat their own disorders by choosing and eating certain grasses and, sometimes, soil (and one can only feel sorry for those whose owners stop them doing so), and horses and other animals choose particular plants, not only grasses, according to their moods and how they are feeling.

The correct term for general plant medicine, as opposed specifically to herbalism, is phytotherapy. Herbs are plants that do not develop persistent, woody tissues above ground level.

There are two main ways in which herbalism works. It provides the body with substances that stimulate the immune system to counteract various disorders, and it is also believed to use substances found in plants to clear the body's energy channels or meridians, allowing its energy to flow freely and in a balanced way again, clearing pathogens ('germs'), toxins and other waste. Both these functions are common to most other complementary therapies as well. They tend to work by stimulating the body to heal itself, whereas orthodox medicine provides drugs that may act as a back-up to the body's own efforts, providing extra substances and effects rather than stimulating the immune system. This is why other therapies are called 'complementary', because they can complement what we now know as orthodox medicine, human or veterinary.

Because of the great interest in complementary therapies, work is being done on several of them to prove how they work, or even that they do work, and this is to the satisfaction of orthodox scientists, doctors and veterinary surgeons. Herbalism is one of the therapies that is known to be effective.

Herbalism was the main therapy in the armoury of healers, including doctors, until around the middle of the 20th century, when the advent of synthetic drugs and antibiotics – the 'big guns' – pushed it into the background. Herbs still form part of modern medicines; for example, aspirin comes from salicylic acid from willow and digitalis (used in heart disease) from foxgloves. However, orthodox medicine still tends to extract what it believes to be the active ingredients from the herbs rather than leaving the herb in its entire state, which has both a balanced and synergistic effect, unlike isolating one ingredient from its 'working partners'. When synthetic forms of the active ingredients are manufactured artificially in a laboratory, often in a concentrated form, both the valuable synergistic and also the regulating or balancing benefits may be lost in the final product. This may be one reason why other undesirable side-effects occur in synthetic medicines.

Herbalism comes under the heading of a holistic, 'natural', complementary or alternative therapy and, as such, in some countries a referral from an orthodox veterinary surgeon is required before being able to consult a medical herbalist for the treatment of your horse in conjunction with or without conventional veterinary treatment. There are, though, countless herbal products from feed supplements to topical medicines (those applied to a particular site on the body) that can readily be bought from feed merchants and tack shops. Feed manufacturers often produce at least one type of feed containing herbs, and some market whole ranges for horses with various problems.

Any therapy is best used in accordance with the advice of a qualified specialist, and herbalism is no different. Unknowledgeable people giving a bit of this supplement and a bit of that may not only fail to achieve the desired effect, but could cause problems through feeding wrong amounts or substances that may not be compatible with each other. Any herbal product must be used strictly in accordance with the directions on its container, and it is wise not to use more than one at a time without the advice of a medical herbalist or nutritionist experienced in herbalism.

I have been fortunate with my veterinary surgeons and have never been refused a referral to a herbalist (or other therapist). However, although the herbalist has always wanted to know what other medicine the animal has been prescribed by its orthodox vet, the vets have very rarely enquired what treatment the herbalist has prescribed. Only one, in many years, has been seriously interested. This is a great shame as I know from my own consistent experience that herbalism can help in various conditions in which orthodox human or animal medicine does poorly. The commonsense way would be for all healers to respect each other and work together.

Whether I have used commercial herb supplements for my horses or been prescribed medicines made up for them by a herbalist, I have never had a horse refuse a feed with the correct amount of a product or medicine in it. Some herbs have quite a strong smell and taste (I use herbalism for myself, too) and you would think that fussy eaters would be put off their feed by them, but I have not found this.

Herbs in Pasture

Sowing a herb strip on the driest part of a paddock is a good idea. It gives horses much more choice of grazing plants and it also gives them the facility to treat themselves naturally, as they would in the wild. Mixing the herbs in with the normal grass plants of the paddock is not normally recommended except for vigorously growing herbs, as the grass may well smother the herbs and prevent them growing. Herbs also will not do well on land that tends to be cold, damp or wet, which is why the driest part is advised to be set aside for herbs.

If you have your own land or have it on lease for a fairly long period, you can sow a herb strip for your horses. Advice should be taken from an agronomist or seed merchant as to which herbs will grow in your paddocks and be useful for horses. A consultation with a qualified herbalist would certainly be a good plan to help decide what herbs to introduce.

Common ailments that horses may wish to treat for themselves include digestive disorders, skin irritations, infestation by parasites (both external and internal) and respiratory problems. It is noticeable how horses eat different plants, not only herbs, at different times of year and in varying conditions of climate and health. This is partly because the plants taste differently at different times of year, but also because horses may develop a taste or craving for a particular nutrient or substance in a given plant, which can treat a minor problem naturally. Therefore, the wider the choice of grazing to which horses have access, the easier it is for them to care for their own health and well-being.

Chapter 10
THE SENSE OF HEARING

Horses have voices, but they are not noisy, very vocal animals. Indeed, spending some time with a herd of horses contentedly grazing and socializing together will result in an observer realizing just how quiet they are with each other. Horses can hear higher-frequency sounds than humans, and their vocalizations may contain high-frequency harmonics, which they can detect and which may be relevant in communication. Humans can hear slightly lower-pitched sounds than horses. Elephants make low rumbling infrasounds, but horses do not appear to make high ultrasounds.

Although their two separate ears can each make a 180-degree semicircle from front to back to help direct sound waves down the ear, horses in general probably cannot pinpoint the source of sound waves very effectively (**41, 42**). As just one example, I kept one of my mares for a while at a yard where one of the paddocks was on top of

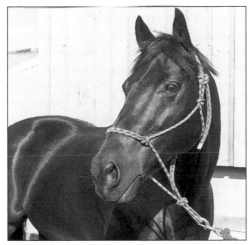 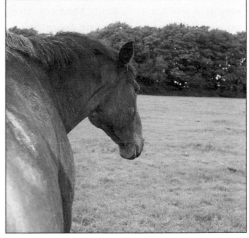

41 The positioning of the ears is a reliable guide to where the horse is directing his attention. This horse is interested in something off to his right and some distance away. His ears are pricked in that direction, his head is up and turned towards it so that he can get a clear view with both eyes in the area of his binocular vision, and his nostrils are open as he tries to take in any smells that might help him to identify whatever it is.

42 Although the photographer is behind this horse, he does not have to move much to keep track of what she is doing. The head is turned just enough for him to see her with his right eye, and his right ear is directed straight towards her. Horses often pay attention to more than one situation at a time by moving their ears independently.

a high, steep bank. This bank was on the far side of a small rural park close to where I lived and where I used to walk my dog. One day, while walking my dog in the park, I could just see my mare grazing near the paddock fence on top of the bank. She had her tail to the fence and, as I climbed the bank, not trying to be particularly quiet, I realized that she could not see me and did not appear to have heard me, either. I reached the fence, by which time she had moved about ten metres away from the fence and was facing directly away from me, her companions being some distance further on. I said her name very quietly. She did hear this. She stopped grazing, but did not lift her head and remained stock still for some seconds, then started grazing again. I said her name again, just a little louder. This time her head swung up but still did not turn, despite the fact that she thought the sound was coming from behind her because her ears were pointed directly back towards me. She stopped chewing and was absolutely still for what seemed like a long time. She was listening intently, but clearly could not see me as I leaned on the fence behind her. Finally, I said her name in a normal tone of voice and she did an amazing manoeuvre for a mare in her twenties. She shot straight up in the air, turned round in mid-air and landed facing me. I have never seen anything like it before or since. She stood rooted to the spot, ears pricked hard towards me, eyes almost on stalks, clearly as amazed at seeing any human in that spot as I was at the feat she had just performed. Yet she did not approach until I spoke to her again. At the sound of my voice, and having me within her range of vision as well, she relaxed and walked over for a chat and a fuss.

As a prey animal by nature, I would have expected her to turn and check on the sound if not the first time, then certainly the second time she heard me speak, as she clearly knew it was coming from behind her and from a completely unaccustomed place. But she didn't. She also did not approach the third time I called her name, despite my having used a normal tone of voice and also her being able to see me by then. We know that horses have rather indistinct eyesight so maybe, at around ten yards, she did not fully recognize me (maybe because she was not expecting to see me) until I spoke to her the fourth time, when she was clearly certain that it was me. Maybe the shock of seeing a human in a place where humans never went contributed to her confusion.

The vocal noises horses make seem fairly limited to most of us, although author and horseman Henry Blake claimed to have differentiated many sounds and variations of them over many years of observation. He described them in his trilogy of books, eventually published in one volume entitled 'Horse Sense'.

THE USE OF VOICE

Voice is a very important and valuable means of communicating with horses, even though they seem, in their own societies, to make little use of their own voices. Horses are certainly very susceptible to the human voice. They can easily distinguish from its tone what mood we are in, whether or not we are pleased, relaxed, nervous, cross, weak, assertive, giving a definite command or request or simply conversing (43, 44). Horses operate best from simple, clear sounds, although they can pick out particular words or short phrases from a general conversation with another human. One example relates to a former circus horse who reared as part of his act. A common command to rear on the circus is 'high'. This caused quite a lot of trouble when people near the horse greeted each other with the word 'Hi', even when they followed it with other words such as 'how are you?'. The horse would rear even though there was no trainer in front of him giving the visual signal to rear (a raised whip in each hand). It was felt best not to confuse the horse by trying to train him out of his long-time habit, instead it was decied not to use the word 'Hi'.

Another example relates to a horse who used to go to his manger every time he heard his owner say the word 'carrots', because this was the word the owner said when she gave him his ration. If she said it in conversation with another person, not even looking at her horse, he would go to his manger expecting his treat to appear.

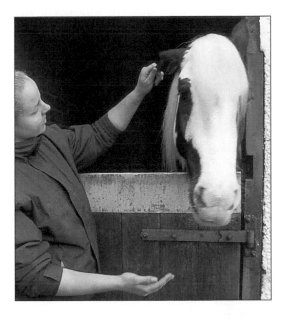

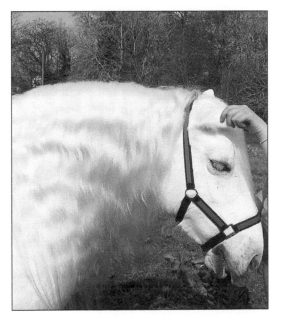

43, 44 (43) Horses respond readily to the tone and level of the human voice, even when a specific command is not being spoken. A few minutes' friendly conversation often reassures them that nothing much is happening and the person is in a good mood. This is also a good way of getting a horse to accept having something done that he does not like, such as having his ears touched, something many horses dislike. (44) On the other hand, gently pulling the ears in your hands, like this, is something some horses really enjoy. This pony clearly likes it, as you can see from the expression on her face.

A Natural Aid

Whether handling, training, riding, driving, working our horses loose or calling them in from the field, the human voice is invaluable and is classified as one of the natural aids. The modern tendency not to use the voice much seems to stem from it not being allowed in most dressage tests, although the UK's Classical Riding Club allows moderate use of it in their tests. It is strange that this recognized, natural aid is banned in competitive dressage, the only sport in which this is done so far as I am aware. The sport stems from military practice, when horses were used at night and had to work to silent aids so as not to be detected by the enemy. Time is long overdue for this now irrelevant rule to be rescinded.

In schooling and training it is so much easier on human and horse to have the latter respond to vocal aids. The standards of traditional, high-level horsemanship of any kind demand:

• Ease of control for safety.
• Willing cooperation, which most horses will give if they understand what is wanted.
• Lightness in the horse due to correct way of going and self-balance.
• Harmony and balance on the rider's part.
• Subtle, even invisible, aids from the rider.

Using the voice to make your requests to a horse means that you can sit there and do less with your seat, legs and reins, concentrating not so much on what the horse is doing but more on how he is doing it, using your voice and physical aids to encourage him to dress himself. The word 'dress' in this context has the original and correct meaning of 'putting the finishing touches to something'. The word 'dressage' does not, strictly speaking, simply mean 'training' or 'schooling'; it also means 'putting the finishing touches' to a horse's actions or performance. For example, a number of soldiers can line up and then may be commanded to 'dress left', thereby making the line straighter as they each shuffle into a better position.

If you ride with a willingness to use your voice readily and effectively, it is relatively easy to maintain an excellent balance in the saddle, thus improving your security, and still have an easily compliant horse – the aim of all skilled and sensitive riders. In any case, a number of competitive dressage riders are really good ventriloquists and give vocal commands or reassurances to their horses through a fixed smile.

Driving horses go largely to the voice, as do circus horses, although in performance the music tends to drown the voice out. This is where they rely not only on the trainer's physical, visual signals, but also on the particular music, which they associate with each movement in their act.

Dr Marthe Kiley-Worthington (Kiley-Worthington, 2005), who is interested in educating her horses rather than just training them, has accustomed her horses to respond to far more words and phrases than most horsemen and women use to their horses. Indeed, most people think that horses do not have the intelligence to understand (link sounds to objects or actions) more than a very basic vocabulary. I am sure that most of us use many different words and phrases to our horses out of a desire to express ourselves to ourselves, not only to our horses, so making ourselves feel better and not really expecting the horse to respond to them and actually do anything.

As an example, take the fairly common scenario of a horse who will not stand still while being groomed or tacked up (45). The owner very often looks at the situation from his or her own viewpoint, not that of the horse, and a vocal tirade such as 'For goodness sake, will you keep still? How many times do I have to tell you?', sometimes accompanied by a slap on the belly or a jab on the reins or lead rope, is the usual result. Although the horse may be able to tell from the tone of voice that the owner is displeased, most horses are unlikely to make the connection between their owner's displeasure and their fidgeting about. It is even worse if the horse has actually been taught to understand that 'stand' means he is to stand still until asked to move, but the owner does not bother with the discipline of saying 'stand' each and every time he or she wants the horse to do so. The owner somehow expects the horse to stand still without being asked (only very experienced horses usually do this), and then loses patience when he moves around because he/she has failed to tell him (by saying 'stand') what is wanted. How confusing must this be to the horse?

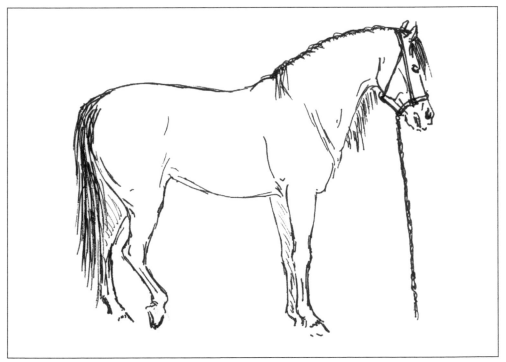

45 Teaching a horse to stand still when his lead rope is simply dropped to the ground (known as ground tying) is really useful. By using the word 'stand' when he is tied to something firm, and positioning him back again whenever he moves, the horse soon learns to stand still. He can gradually progress to being tied to a tree trunk on the ground, to a lighter branch or pole and eventually to nothing. It is important not to leave the horse alone while he is learning this technique.

This general way of communicating is very common in all sorts of situations. The rider/handler feels better because he/she has told the horse off and vented his/her displeasure on the cause of it, the 'naughty' horse, but he/she has done nothing to correct the situation, which could be done by simply saying 'stand' firmly and quietly, assuming that the horse knows what this means. Sometimes, when I am teaching, I come across a rider who will say rather sarcastically to her horse when he is doing something unwanted or resisting (or whatever), 'Er, thank you very much, do you mind?', which, of course, is absolutely useless as a reprimand or correction to any animal. Even worse is when an owner hits the horse because he does not amend his behaviour in response to what has been said. This may make the owner feel better, maybe even good, but it does not achieve the aim of correcting the horse's behaviour.

It is more effective by far, when communicating vocally with a horse, to keep the word or phrase short and always the same. It is also very effective to vary the tone of voice from strict to friendly depending on how familiar the horse is with the words being used and the actual circumstances. For instance, in the example given above of a horse not standing still, if he is a young horse not confirmed in standing still, he should be put back where he was and, when he is still, say 'stand' in a clear and firm but not abrasive tone. The horse can then associate 'stand' with standing still. This can be followed by 'good boy' in a pleased tone and a stroke low down on the neck or withers (46). If he is a very experienced horse, 'stand' spoken in a quiet, friendly tone is usually enough to get him to do so. If this same experienced horse knows he is expected to stand but walks around, put him back where he was and command 'stand' in a firmer tone. He will certainly understand, but, having a mind of his own, this does not mean that he will comply!

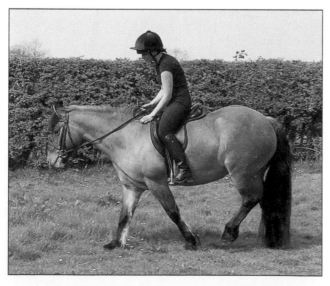

46 Stroking and rubbing horses in the area of the lower neck, below the withers and just behind them, is known to calm them down and actually lower the heart rate. The horse will soon associate a kindly spoken word accompanying this feeling with relaxation and the knowledge that his rider or handler is calm and everything is alright. Then, when riding, the actual movement can be dispensed with, if necessary, and just the spoken word used.

Shouting

It is always said that we should never shout at a horse and, in general, this is certainly true. I do not shout at horses close to me unless being attacked. Like any freelance teacher, I come across all sorts of horses and sometimes you just have to defend yourself. The trick is to make your reprimand a short, sharp and unmistakable one, and then to change your demeanour like lightning, because in a few seconds the horse may well have moved on mentally and not deserve a reprimand at that moment. The horse must connect the reprimand with his action at the time. After two seconds, behavioural trainers tell us, a horse cannot mentally make the connection between our vocal sound and his action. I am not entirely convinced of this, but bow to specialist opinion in this case and follow that advice. It certainly works.

In my opinion, a quiet or louder growling sound is a very good corrective. I like the word 'no' as a general corrective, said in different tones of voice. A very quiet 'no' is enough for a familiar horse who surely understands it and is usually cooperative. With others who are not in the habit of cooperating (usually because they have not been taught to, but occasionally because of their nature), a firmer, louder 'no' is needed and if that does not work, a good growl usually does.

Once the horse has stopped doing whatever it was that elicited the 'no' or growl, the vocal aids must be stopped and the horse praised for doing the right thing, usually by saying something like 'yes' or 'good girl' in a pleased tone and by stopping/releasing any physical aids that you were also giving. Some behavioural trainers believe that horses do not understand reward as such; they merely associate the release or stopping of an aid or vocal command with their new action (doing what the handler or rider wanted). However, based on my experience, I do not agree with this viewpoint. I am certain that horses do understand very well when we are pleased with them or vice versa by our tone of voice and demeanour.

A Suggested Human–Equine Vocabulary

The words and phrases I have found essential as a basic vocabulary are few but comprehensive. Firstly, the horse's name; it is a great attention getter and the first thing professional show-business horses are taught. I use a horse's name before giving any vocal request if the horse appears at all distracted; for example, 'Rose, over' or 'Rose, back'. When riding, it is also good to use the horse's name before asking for something, particularly on an inexperienced or partly schooled horse, provided you know that he does connect your vocal sound with the action you want.

The other words that horses should understand and which form a minimal vocabulary are 'no', 'yes' or 'good boy', 'stand', 'foot up' (for picking out feet), 'back', 'over', 'walk on', 'trot on' or 'terr-ot' (as they both sound quite different, decide which one you want to use), 'can-ter', 'easy' (for calming down) and, perhaps, the traditional 'whoa' for slowing down. Some people also use 'whoa' for stopping, even though they also use 'stand'. Horses seem able to differentiate between 'whoa' for slowing down and stopping from movement and 'stand' to keep them still. In Iberia, a long drawn-out 'aaaaah' is used to indicate the cessation of something or a short rest, and the horses slow and relax at once.

To a horse all these are just noises or sounds. The language in which a horse is trained means nothing to him, only the sound. Imported horses soon learn the language of their new homeland and many who are moved around a country and experience different accents get used to them in fairly quick order. An example of this was a Morgan stallion imported to England who would not canter on the lunge for his English handler until she said the command with a strong American accent. The poor horse, who was amenable and a perfect gentleman, must have been quite anxious when being given repeatedly a command he just didn't understand. Another Thoroughbred stallion tried to attack anyone with a Geordie accent (from north-east England), as he had been in training there and obviously had bad memories involving that distinctive accent.

Teaching Commands or Vocal Aids

Most people who purchase horses buy ready backed and, often, trained horses. Some people do buy unbacked youngsters with very basic training, used to at least walking in hand, stopping and standing, having their bodies handled and, it is hoped, a very basic vocabulary. Few people buy completely unhandled, green or even wild horses who know no words whatsoever. Working on this basis, you do at least have a foundation on which to start. Foals should be taught basic handling on the stud, although only the bigger and better studs with adequate staff seem to sell youngstock with this training today because of the time and financial costs of employing suitable labour.

Assuming that your new horse understands a few words, it is important to use them readily in order to get him used to you and your specific, chosen commands. As you begin to lead him and he moves off say 'walk on', so that he associates the movement (walking) with the command. When he does make this association, you can simply say the command and he will (should!) walk. The same with trotting; as he trots in hand, on the lunge or under saddle in response to your physical aids say immediately 'trot on', so that he comes to realize that that particular sound accompanies trotting. The command should then produce a trot once the penny has dropped.

Many people find that horses do not clearly understand the command to canter. The way to get a horse to canter on the lunge (on large circles only), if he does not know the command, is to send him on in a trot that is a little too fast for comfort, and the instant he breaks into canter say 'can-ter – good boy' in a really pleased tone, so that he associates the sound with the action. After just a few strides bring him back to trot by saying the command of your choice – perhaps 'whoa' then 'trot on'. Depending on the horse and his or her temperament, do not canter a horse unused to it for more than a few strides at first in case he starts regarding it as an excuse to start bucking and kicking. As his strength and balance improve he increasingly can do a little more. A low, soothing sound has the effect of relaxing and slowing down a horse and a more brightly spoken one chirps him up and sends him on.

As a teacher, I find that jogging alongside a ridden horse and saying the command in a bright tone and occasionally carefully clapping my hands certainly gets them to lift up in their present or a new gait, although I once did this and the horse quite unexpectedly went into a bucking fit, throwing his rider. I felt dreadful, but the rider thought it was funny! I have been much more careful since.

Your body position when lunging also helps. Standing level with the horse's hip at a slight angle to his head and facing the way he is going sends him on, whereas standing level with his shoulder and facing slightly away from the direction of movement slows him down. The use of the whip is also important. Pointed at his hindquarters it should send him on, but pointed at or in front of his head should help to slow him down.

A word about lunging in general. A serious and very common fault in conventional lunging is to keep the line 'reeled' in with several loops in the hand and, therefore, quite short, forcing the horse on to much too small a circle. Small circles are an advanced movement under saddle and are very difficult under any kind of constraint (which covers lunging) for any but a correctly muscled-up, experienced horse (47). The lunge line is the length it is for a reason – to give the horse a comfortable amount of ground to go on a circle without being forced to go incorrectly and out of balance. This will not only develop the wrong muscles, but also possibly strain soft tissues and joints. It will also do nothing for the horse's view of his work, leading to dislike and possible evasions. The rein should be let out to almost its full length very quickly during a lunging session, unless the horse is larking about and you need to control and settle him before starting work. It is also not a good idea to stand rigidly in the centre of the circle, determinedly rooted to the spot. Circle work is difficult and tiring, so be prepared to walk with the horse and perform plenty of ovals and straight lines as well as circles, using the whole of your schooling area for interest.

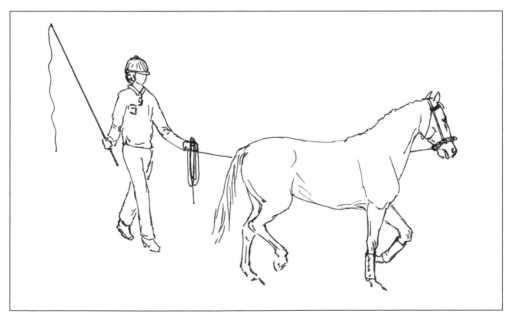

47 This is a common picture when horses are being lunged. Lunging on too short a rein, forcing small circles, is very difficult for any but very supple horses, causing them to become unbalanced.

The key to teaching commands is to say the word as the horse performs the action, so that he associates the two together and eventually the command alone makes it clear to him what you want, even if you need a physical aid as backup. Saying it beforehand, such as telling the horse to pick his 'foot up' before he does so, will produce no result and may worry him slightly, as he knows you want something but does not know what.

Training and discipline (essential for safety of both humans and horses) should begin almost as soon as a foal is born. On a good, responsible stud/stud farm, a foal is taught the command 'walk on' from day 2 by someone holding and leading the dam and another person, possibly two, gently restraining the foal with an arm or two arms around his neck and a stable rubber or another arm behind his hindquarters. As the dam's handler walks her on, the foal will follow and his handler gently pushes him from behind and says 'walk on'. The restraint from the front end controls the foal's speed and actions (no leaping forwards or up in the air). When the dam and foal reach the paddock gate or the other side of the stable, whatever is their destination, the restraint comes gently but firmly from the front end against the foal's chest, accompanied by the command 'stand'. In a very few days the commands alone are enough, combined with consistent firm and gentle physical restraint or encouragement, to produce a well-behaved foal who not only watches his dam and follows her example, but also listens to and obeys his handlers. In this way, horses learn from their earliest days to obey general, necessary vocal aids.

TONIC IMMOBILITY

Tonic immobility is a condition first described by the late Dr Moyra Williams and by several other people, including members of the EBF and this author, some years ago. The condition is one in which a horse will suddenly stop and become rooted to the spot, and become completely oblivious to everything in his immediate environment. The horse will be in a state of high alertness and be tense, but not at all frightened; indeed, he may seem quite relaxed but apparently completely unaware of his surroundings, totally absorbed in some distant phenomenon that his rider or handler cannot detect. This is not the same state as that normally described as catatonic immobility, in which animals, and people, are paralysed by fear and simply cannot move.

All the horses described appeared to be 'tuned in' to some kind of communication reaching them from afar. Their heads would be high, their eyes wide, their nostrils flared and their ears hard pricked directly in front of them. They would gaze off into the far distance but, although clearly not in any kind of trance, did not appear to be looking at anything specific. They would look around and, although their nostrils would be flared, they did not sniff the air or seem to be sensing any kind of aroma. They all gave every impression of, as one member put it, 'receiving a message from outer space' or some other dimension. There was no sign of fear or even apprehension in any of them, just rapt attention on something far away. Despite the state of tension in their bodies, affected horses gave no sign of being about to take to their heels in the typical flight response to something frightening.

Another interesting point about the condition was that no matter what their riders or handlers did to get them to move on, none of of the horses would budge an inch, or even move a foot. In fact, the horses did not seem to be aware of their human companions at all and some owners said they tried using fairly strong inducements to get their horses to move, without any success. We were all powerless to do anything about the situation and just had to wait until the horses snapped out of it, which they did after a couple of minutes, continuing on their way as if nothing had happened.

Looking back, I now feel sure that the horses were listening to something far away that clearly they could detect, but which was outside the range of human hearing. We know that horses can hear sounds of a higher frequency than people and from farther away, so this could certainly be an explanation and it fits all the symptoms shown by the horses described.

One aspect of the condition that I cannot explain is that nothing the owners of these horses did would induce them to move. One owner said she gave her horse a couple of hefty blows with her whip to get him out of it because they were on a fairly busy road when he went into this condition, but he gave no reaction at all. Once, when my own horse did it (one of several times in different places) we were on a bridleway with a tractor, a couple of farm dogs and a herd of cattle slowly bearing down on us from some way behind, but my horse nevertheless stopped dead and focused all his attention on another orbit. Although I was becoming panic stricken because my horse did not like cattle, he seemed to have forgotten they were there. Miraculously, he came back down to earth before they quite reached us (not because of them, I am certain) and we escaped, at a calm walk, down another route.

Some owners said they had thought it was only their own horse who demonstrated this condition and that they had described it to friends, who passed it off as weird. Others said they did not dare tell anyone about it in case people thought they were crazy or had done something awful to their horse. How relieved they were to find it reported in the EBF's journal, *Equine Behaviour*.

MUSIC AS THERAPY AND RELAXATION – OR OTHERWISE

The effects of music on horses can be quite marked, even though it is a completely unnatural experience for them. My own observations and those of other people are that they like soft, 'easy listening' music, relaxing and inspiring classical music, military music, and recordings of natural sounds like birdsong and running water. Highly-strung horses can certainly be calmed down by quiet, relaxing music played in short spells of, say, twenty minutes at a time. It is known to increase the appetite and milk yield in dairy cows coming in for milking, and my observations are that it can calm horses as well.

Classical master, the late Nuno Oliveira, usually had appropriate classical music playing while he worked his horses, as did my own teacher of the 1980s, Desi Lorent, who trained with Oliveira. Horses definitely enjoy carefully chosen music and work well to it, often producing extra élan and style. Circus horses live with music in their work, and they remember particular tunes for many years, associating them with the acts they used to perform. I have seen some circus horses clearly enjoying performing movements to music, without cues from a trainer, years later.

I once had an ex-race mare who used to prance around her box every time she heard the local silver band. If she was out in the field, she would passage up and down the fence. She also became very excited and hard to handle when my husband and I were leading her down to the local show one year, to the extent that we had to bring her home again. It is possible that it reminded her of the excitement of the racecourse, but this same mare hated music playing on a radio in the stable yard and used to weave continually until it was turned off, as did another Thoroughbred gelding I had.

There is no doubt that horses can become very agitated and troubled by loud music of any kind (not surprising in view of their sensitive hearing), and appear particularly to dislike rock and similar music and unmelodious music, and also human voices on radio talk programmes and violins (my findings). It always surprises and concerns me (for the horses) that so many people leave radios on in the stables more or less all the time, even when they themselves are not listening to them and regardless of what sounds are coming out of them. It is not difficult for any reasonably sensitive person to feel the tension coming from the horses and to see their distress in these circumstances. I have often gone to teach people and actually had to ask them to turn the radio off while we discussed something or had a lesson.

Some horses start performing stereotypical actions (stable vices) under these circumstances (e.g. box walking, weaving, head tossing and twirling, crib biting, wind sucking and kicking walls and doors). They may also stop eating, get up if lying down and generally look stressed and upset.

What many people overlook is that horses are absolute prisoners in their boxes. Not only can they not turn the din off or even down, they cannot even tell someone to do it for them unless that someone is actually present and is perceptive enough to recognize how disturbed the horses are. Some yards, run by people who really should know better, believe that the radio provides company for the horses when there are no humans present. The last thing a horse wants is the sound of human voices all the time or music constantly playing or blaring randomly out of a radio. One yard I know plays the radio in the barn 24 hours a day. Obviously, in circumstances such as those described above, run by people who can only be described as selfish and insensitive, music, far from being therapeutic, is nothing but psychological torture. Advertisements are appearing in animal magazines for CDs featuring music and sound effects that are claimed to heal, calm and relax animals. These could be well worth trying, but it would be advisable to watch your horse closely to make sure that he or she is really responding to them, or to any music, as you wish.

BALANCE

Balance is the general equilibrium of the body. It is controlled from the cerebrum or front part of the brain, mainly receiving its stimuli from the semicircular canals in the ears, but also in response to stimuli from the feet, limbs and eyes.

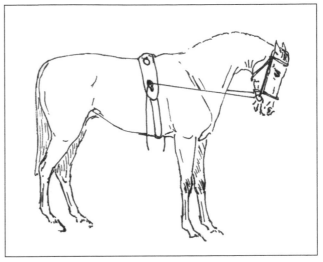

48 Some people still use harsh methods to try to get their horses and ponies to adopt what they believe is a 'correct' position or body posture, with the head forced in at an unnatural angle. This drawing shows a pony left standing in his stable with his head tied into such a position. This is an ineffective way of achieving their aim, because good posture and a correctly developed physique can only come from logical gymnastic work that does not involve the use of force. The practice shown here causes pain and stiffness in the body due to unrelieved tension. It does not 'make a horse accept the bit', but causes him to resent and evade it, and is surely an altogether unacceptable practice on the grounds of equine welfare.

Transport

When the semicircular canals receive and detect unusual or unnatural movement or vibration, the fluid disturbance in the canals is thought to create a sense of loss of balance. It is known that many animals experience travel sickness, so horses probably do as well. This is probably one of the many reasons why horses do not wish to travel in trailers or horseboxes. It seems that in large horseboxes, horses travelling above or behind the rear wheels experience the most uncomfortable movements and vibrations and probably experience the most distress and travel sickness when in transit. It would seem a good plan to use this area for transporting equipment and feed instead of horses.

Jumping

Because the ears are the main means of maintaining equilibrium, it is important not to unreasonably restrict the horse's head carriage when it is being ridden. (Another reason is the horse's vision, which is dealt with in the next chapter on the Sense of Sight.) It is commonly taught that the horse's head and neck are his balancing pole, equivalent to our arms in our more extreme movements such as running, jumping and general athletic movements, yet many people do not allow their horse to use them. Indeed, they purposely restrict the horse's use of his head and neck in what they see as being in the interest of control (48). If the skill was used and time was taken to properly school and habituate a horse to cooperating with the rider's aids, this kind of control would not be necessary. Instead we frequently see horses 'fighting for their heads' in an effort to balance themselves properly and see where they are going. The more the horse struggles the harder and harsher is the rider's pressure via the bit on the horse's mouth. Stronger and stronger bits are used, hoisted too high in the horse's mouth, nosebands are cranked tighter and tighter, and various kinds of training aids and control devices are used to try to ensure control. Jumping (and other activities) becomes a battle, or at least a serious argument, between horse and rider instead of the beautiful, calm, quiet picture it can be of a skilled, sensitive rider and a properly trained, confident, trusting horse.

Particularly when horses are jumping, it is noticeable that many riders do not allow them a free head when in flight over obstacles. This must in some measure affect the horse's sensory experience of his own movements when trying to negotiate his fences. How does a horse jump when left to his own devices? As he approaches a fence he will slightly lower his head and neck to bring the obstacle into focus onto the retina at the back of his eyes, then raise them along with the forehand and bring them very slightly back as he lifts his forehand in take-off. Immediately after this, as his body rises into the air, he will stretch his head and neck out, forward and down over the fence, balancing himself perfectly in a classic bascule or arc, which is a very beautiful, natural movement to watch. On landing, he brings the head and neck up and back a little before continuing on his way.

Unfortunately, what often happens in riding is that riders strongly restrict the position of the horse's head and neck in the approach in an effort to control his speed and/or get him to adjust his stride and take off at the right spot, or where the rider tells him (not always the same thing!). The rider should, at least, immediately release the head and neck as the forehand leaves the ground and the head and neck, having come back a little, then start to go forward to 'round' over the fence. What happens very often at this moment is that the rider pulls back on the reins with his or her hands, not only preventing the head and neck from moving forward, but actually pulling them backward. This basically is caused by the rider trying to keep his or her balance because of having an insufficiently secure seat, which depends on balance, over fences. Riders can then often be seen to lean forward and push their hands up the crest of the horse's neck towards the ears to 'give him his head'. This often causes the lower leg to move backwards along the horse's sides, which adds to the insecurity of the seat or riding position. Also, the hands being up on the crest of the neck often provide a convenient support for the rider to lean on for stability, which should not be necessary. Although this weight on the horse's neck is, in itself, unlikely to influence the head and neck to go down too much and upset the horse's natural balance even more, it does mean that the classic straight line from the elbow, through the hand, down the rein to the horse's mouth is destroyed. The shortest route between two points is always a straight line, so holding the hands up the neck produces an inverted V-shape from the elbow, up to the hands and down to the horse's mouth, effectively 'shortening' the reins, reducing the distance to the horse's mouth and creating or increasing a contact on it at just the time when the horse needs the exact opposite (i.e freedom of the head and neck).

In previous decades, the sought after jumping seat, which was developed during the latter part of the 19th century and, particularly, the first half of the 20th century, and used in high-level competition over massive fences with great success up to the late 1980s, was as follows:

- The horse and rider canter (or trot, if the jumps are fairly low to moderate in height) towards the jump. The rider's shoulders are just above his knees or slightly behind them and his lower leg is more or less vertically below his thigh. If he looked down he could probably just see the toe of his boot. His weight is allowed to drop straight down into his heel and his stirrup leathers (on a suitably designed, fairly forward-cut jumping saddle, with forward-set stirrup bars over which the stirrup leathers hang) are vertical from the stirrup bars downwards. His hands, holding the reins, are on the straight line – elbow, hand, horse's mouth – and he has a light, guiding but ideally non-restrictive feel or contact on the horse's mouth, the horse being well-schooled and, therefore, confident enough not to rush his fences. Depending on the type of fence being jumped, the horse will, it is hoped, be in a powerful but moderately fast canter, not pulling his rider's arms out, producing plenty of energy and impulsion from his engine (his hindquarters) and, most importantly, travelling within his own balance, not relying on being 'held up' in any way by his rider. (This is not a counsel of perfection; it used to happen regularly, and rather more than it appears to do today.)
- On approaching the fence, in an effort to retain a light, elastic contact with the horse's mouth, the rider adopts a 'following' feel with his hands, adapting to the position of his horse's mouth rather than vice versa. So, when the horse raises his head a little on take-off, the rider's hands will come back a little towards his body and his upper body starts to fold down as if he is trying to touch the horse's crest with his breastbone, rather than leaning, or lurching, forward. The lower leg remains vertical for security of balance and position, not swinging backwards or, even worse, unless it is a drop fence, forwards.
- The horse's critical movement of the head and neck is now to stretch forwards, out and down as he bascules over the fence in his natural jumping movement. The rider, sitting still, quiet and folded down from the hips, allows his hands to be taken passively forwards and down with and towards the horse's mouth, not pushing them up towards his ears in a mistaken belief that he is 'lifting' the horse over the fence (clearly impossible) or giving him freedom of his head (which is best achieved with the straight line/hands following technique). In practice, the hands follow the horse's mouth and will actually travel forwards diagonally down the shoulders, maintaining the shortest route of the elbow/hand/horse's mouth straight line, so giving the horse maximum freedom of his head and neck. Sometimes it is necessary to let the reins run through the fingers somewhat if the fence is a wide spread or the horse stands back and takes off a little early. Both these techniques give the horse every chance to make his best, unrestricted effort to clear his fence.
- As he descends from the maximum height he has reached over the obstacle, the horse's head and neck start to come up and back again, as does the rider's upper body. The hands maintain the light contact on the horse's mouth by coming back towards the upper body and, as the horse completes his landing, the rider's upper body resumes its previous, pre-jump position to help the horse in his getaway. The horse has jumped as freely as possible and the rider has made as little interfering movement as possible, staying in quiet balance, simply folding down and up again by means of mainly his hip joints and giving the horse his head by following down and forwards with his hands.

This is a perfect jump from horse and rider (49–51), but it is by no means an unreachable ideal. Jumps were just as high and wide in show jumping and cross-country competitions of the past, often more so, and they still are in the hunting field. If riders and horses spent more time perfecting their techniques at lower heights (whether for competition or not), they would be able to tackle bigger fences in better balance and, surely, more safely than often seems to be the case today. Fashions change in everything and it would be good to see the pendulum swing back towards this more stylish, better balanced and less interfering way of riding. The better the balance, the more chance the horse has of not only jumping more successfully, but of enjoying the experience and, surely, of trying harder, rider permitting.

With some of the more restrictive styles of riding seen, done by the rider partly to keep his or her balance on top and partly in an effort to control the horse, the rider is, when looked at in the light of the above description, actively reducing the horse's chances of successfully negotiating his obstacle. Horses can be seen lurching the forehand, head and neck up and back as they approach, jumping with the head in the air or frantically trying to throw it forward in order to gain their balance to jump more naturally. This must move the fluid in the balance mechanism (the semicircular canals) more than if the head was moved naturally during a jump and kept comparatively still. Fighting for his head must disorientate the horse somewhat. This is surely not the best state to be in when jumping. The stillness of a horse's head is a feature of horses jumping loose or freely on the lunge, and it is the first thing to go when an interfering type of rider gets on board.

Restricting and unnaturally influencing the head and neck result in poor jumping technique and use of the horse's body, so he cannot use it to best effect. This can result in lost competitions, stumbles, knocked down fences, falls of horse and rider, particularly if riding over fixed fences, loss of enjoyment and loss of confidence, plus the more serious factors of injuries and even fatalities. Any horse and rider can get things wrong, can miss a stride, let nervousness or even fear affect their actions and have an accident as a result. By working more in a still, balanced way over lower fences to establish confidence and technique, the chances of this happening are reduced.

I should love to see riding that forces the horse to move his head, neck and body in an unnatural way incur faults or penalties in jumping competitions. This would go a long way towards improving riding style and technique, as would more competitions that are actually judged on good style.

Flat Work

A mark of a well-schooled horse is that he travels and performs his movements in self-balance, with guidance from but not restriction by his rider. This has always been the standard of an educated horse and a skilful, empathetic rider. Mutual, harmonious balance between the two is essential for this level of achievement but, sadly, today it often takes a back seat.

As a teacher and trainer, I have ridden and schooled horses who have undergone what seems to be common, conventional training and yet found them without exception initially heavy in hand and relying on me to hold their heads up and in. They are at first incapable of balancing themselves under a rider (something they can

49–51 (49) Diagram showing perfectly balanced position of horse and rider over a jump. The rider is folding the torso down, is not leaning on the horse's neck, is maintaining the straight line from elbow to hand to horse's mouth, and the hands are moving forward and down with the horse's mouth, maintaining the lightest contact to give him complete freedom to stretch over his obstacle while remaining in touch. The line shows the three points of a balanced, independent seat (i.e. shoulder, knee, toe), which should all be on a straight line. (50) A good rider trying this style of jumping for the first time. Her lower legs are down correctly, but instead of folding down her upper body she has leant too far forward. Although she has a straight line from the elbow through the hand to the horse's mouth, she is steadying herself on the horse's neck by leaning on her hands. This fixes the rein and prevents him stretching out his head and neck over the jump. (51) A later attempt sees the rider still too far forward, but her legs are down and stable and she has given the horse complete freedom of his head and neck to enable him to stretch as much as he wants to over this little spread. Some would criticise the loss of contact, but this is far better than fixing the hands on the horse's neck, restricting the rein and depriving the horse of the free use of his natural balancing pole, his head and neck.

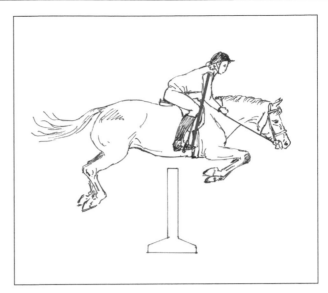

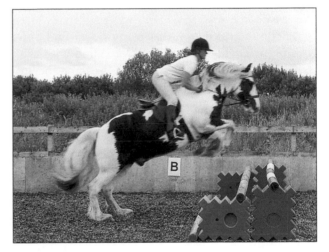

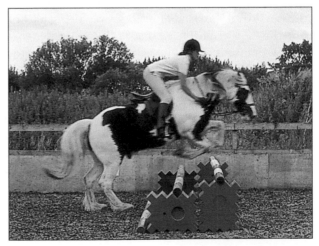

all do easily when at liberty in their fields) but gradually, little by little, I release my hold until they are working comfortably on a friendly, hand holding contact on the outside rein and a light, communicative touch on the inside one. This can be achieved within a few minutes. The next stage is for the horse to be able to work in a suitable posture for his stage of training in self-balance, responding to my seat, so that my hands are no longer his crutch, but another means of light communication.

During work on the flat, the semicircular canals in the ears, which are so instrumental to the horse's balance, do not experience the extent of movement of the head seen in jumping, unless the horse starts cavorting around and bucking. However, the canals are sensitive to even slight movements, and it is more productive and fairer for the horse to have full use of them in all kinds of riding. This is not possible when his head is held in a vice by the rider.

Once a horse has learned a degree of self-balance under a rider who can also balance himself/herself in the saddle, progress can be rapid. The aim is for the horse to concentrate mainly on the rider's seat, thigh and weight aids, although the voice, too, is invaluable, as described earlier. Where the rider puts his/her seat and weight the horse will go; it should not be the other way round – the horse taking the rider for a ride in every sense.

A common situation that many riders find difficult to remedy, because they have not been taught the rudiments of riding with the seat, is the potentially dangerous manoeuvre colloquially known as 'banking' or 'motorbiking', in which the horse, in canter, leans into his bend or circle and usually travels too far in off the rider's desired track. The rider, not unreasonably, leans in with the horse in the belief that she is 'going with the horse', a neat phrase that implies that the rider is a sympathetic horseperson who rides 'as one' with his/her horse. Going with the horse is fine if the horse is going where, and how, you want him to go, but in a case like banking, he is not. Furthermore, 'going with' the horse makes things worse and throws him even more off balance than he already is. Horse and rider are sliding down a very uncomfortable, slippery slope, figuratively speaking.

Why does it happen? Firstly, we need to understand that horses naturally often balance when turning at speed by leading with the inside shoulder and leaning on it, at the same time usually turning the head and neck (the equine balancing pole) to the outside of the bend (a bend simply being part of a circle). Secondly, where a rider puts his/her weight, her horse will go in order to stay in balance. Banking happens for two reasons: 1) the horse is cantering rather too fast for the size of turn or circle being attempted under weight in his present stage of ability, so has to adopt the posture described above; and 2) the rider, already a top-heavy weight on his back, which he tries to balance in order to stay on his feet, destabilizes the horse/rider unit by leaning into the bend, which puts his/her weight to the inside, forcing the horse to travel even further in to stay under the rider and not fall over, although in a bad enough example the pair may well come down. Often, the rider instinctively pulls on the outside rein as well, to ask the horse to move out. This clearly makes things worse, though, as his head is already to the outside, this simply throws even more weight onto the inside shoulder. (Notice a stunt horse falling on to his side – the aid is a pull on the rein away from the side onto which the fall is planned.)

How can all this be corrected? Firstly, the rider needs to slow down the horse with his/her seat, mind and voice and also pulses on the inside rein, which will also have the effect of asking the head to come back to the inside. The seat must be kept still and firm and the upper body upright, and you should keep thinking 'SLOW' to the horse and telling him verbally to slow down, using whatever word he understands. Secondly, the rider also needs to get the horse out onto the required track, not leaning in, and flexing/bending in the direction of the turn or circle. Some weight should be put onto the outside seat bone, down the outside leg and into the outside stirrup; remember, where you put your weight your horse will go. You should also look to the outside of your circle, as where you look is also a powerful directional aid. These actions, combined with having slowed the horse down, will make a rapid, major improvement. The horse has moved out to balance himself up under the rider's weight and is moving slowly enough to be able to control his body. Now the rider can ask for inside flexion with the inside rein and support the horse with the inside leg, particularly the thigh, which is part of the seat. The outside rein controls the speed should the horse speed up again, and the outside leg rests slightly back against the horse's side, preventing the hindquarters swinging out. Problem solved and well done.

The whole point about balance in riding is to keep your own centre of balance as close as possible to that of your horse. If you think of your own as the Centre or Hara of eastern modalities and philosophies, inside your abdomen just below your navel, and that of your horse as inside his thorax/chest cavity about two thirds of the way down and about a hand's width behind his elbow line, and ride so that the two are as close as possible all the time, you will not go far wrong. This clearly means no lurching yourself out of the saddle when jumping any more than you absolutely have to, and no getting 'in front of the movement' or, indeed, behind it when you can possibly avoid it. Think of the two centres like strong magnets constantly pulling towards each other to restore stability, because stability is what you both seek. Stability means security, confidence, safety and partnership – qualities you both want.

Chapter 11
THE SENSE OF SIGHT

Like many creatures, a horse's vision falls short in some ways of that of humans and, especially, birds, but in others he has advantages. We have seen in chapter 6 how the horse's eye is structured and how this affects the way the eye works and the horse's perception of his surroundings (52). Behaviourally, horses do not seem to be significantly less responsive to potential predators in their visual field.

The allocation of rods and cones, respectively the light- and colour-sensitive nerve cells on his retina, indicate that a horse probably sees well in dim light. The horse's colour vision is almost certainly dichromatic. He can probably discern reds and oranges at the red end of the spectrum and violets and blues at the blue end. He may be able to discern yellows and greens in the middle part of the spectrum, but this may not be discernible from white or grey of the same lightness. In all dichromats there will be a wavelength (colour) that cannot be discriminated from white/grey – the dichromatic neutral point. Macuda and Timney (2000) found this to lie at about 480nm in the horse. It is a blue-green colour, so it is not surprising that horses are not able to discriminate colours (e.g. greens) close to this wavelength. The further away from the neutral point the colour lies, the easier, in theory, it is for the horse to discriminate it from a grey of the same lightness.

The horse also sees fairly well in a vertically narrow panorama almost all around his body, mainly monocularly, but with a significant binocular area in front of his head. He cannot see directly behind him when his head is facing straight forward, but a very slight tilt of the head brings into view anything in that area, which he can then see with one eye. Horses have good stereopsis and are good at assessing the two different views

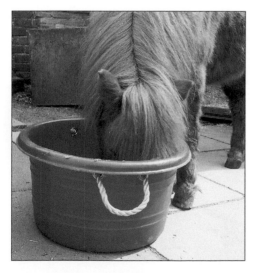

52 Some horses feel insecure about putting their heads into a container deep enough to obscure their vision. This Shetland Pony has no such qualms, being secure in his home environment and only really being interested in food.

presented to them by each individual eye at the same time. There is a blind area in front of the horse's forehead in an upward direction for a distance of something less than about two yards. If a horse wants to bring near objects onto his visual streak of clearest vision, running horizontally along the lower part of his retina just below its equator, he will normally rotate his eyes (which appears to be an involuntary control of eye movement, most of the time) to keep the visual streak horizontal. (The exception is when he tries to look at objects in the sky or above his head. Only then will he voluntarily rotate his eyes so that the iris is no longer horizontal.) However, when a horse tries by this means to look at near objects, he cannot see straight ahead as well and probably his side vision is also reduced.

There is another axis of rotation that corresponds to a horse looking more to the left or the right (or more forward or backward). If a horse is actively attending to an object of curiosity, he will typically rotate his head so that it is pointing at the object and the object is focused on the retinas of both eyes, presumably where it is available to binocular vision and depth perception. If the horse is afraid of an object, he may turn his body away in preparation for flight and look at the object with one eye. If the object is so close as to disappear into the blind spot in front of the horse's face, he will have to turn his head slightly to bring it into view in one eye or the other. All this supposes that the horse has free use of his head and neck, which, when working, he may not have (53–55).

53–55 (53) With the head held at a natural angle for observing something in the mid to far distance, the horse can see ahead, to the side and behind him, below the lines. (54) With the head held in what is commonly regarded as a correct position for 'school' riding, the horse's frontal vision is reduced. (55) This extremely flexed position demanded by some riders clearly greatly reduces the horse's frontal vision to the point of effectively blinding him to what is ahead. (The visual fields shown in all three of these diagrams are a close approximation to the situation in reality.)

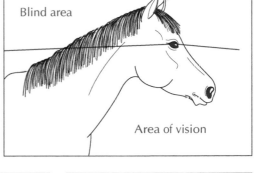

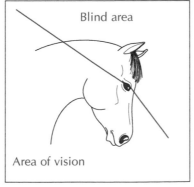

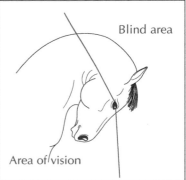

The horse has perfectly good vision for the type of animal he is – a grazing, social, herbivorous, running prey animal (56). With his long head down grazing, he can see his food (grass) well enough to select it with the help of his senses of touch and smell, and also see where to put his feet, which represent security in a galloping prey animal. A horse's ability to detect the tiniest movement much better than humans and almost all around his body (indeed all around his body with a slight turn of the head to either side [57]) gives him excellent early warning of lurking predators, as does his similar ability to detect shape. If he does not spot them, some other herd member, or another species of animal whose body language and alarm calls the Equidae have learnt, invariably will. (Wild and feral Equidae are usually captured by predators when galloping away from them, not by being surprised and leapt upon during grazing.) The horse cannot detect sharp detail, but he does not need to do so for the lifestyle he has evolved to live in nature.

HANDLING AND GROUND WORK

In general, it is important to remember that a horse's vision is less distinct than ours and that he is programmed by his evolution to run away from anything he thinks is suspect. This means giving him the benefit of the doubt when working with and around him. When any apparently suspect objects are causing a horse concern, you should initially place yourself between them and him as protection and as an example that you are not afraid. If you already have a good relationship with your horse, he will probably trust you not to lead him into danger and will follow you past. As he

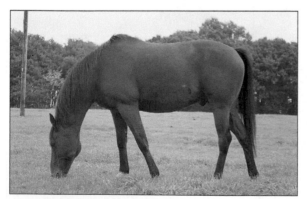

56 Perfect structure for a grazing, running animal. When the head is down, the horse's eyes are raised above the ground and his more or less all-round view is barely obstructed by his relatively thin legs.

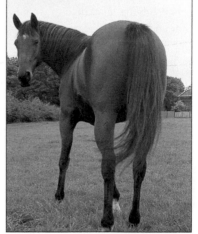

57 Without having to move a foot, the horse can bring into view anything behind him by just turning his very flexible neck.

gains confidence over time, he should accept your word that everything is fine and go past without much objection or anxiety. Trusted people on the ground are a great help when dealing with horses. Horses gain confidence and 'moral support' from them and they can help the trainer if things go wrong.

Ground work can include lunging (58, 59), long reining (60, 61) and various

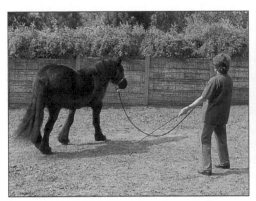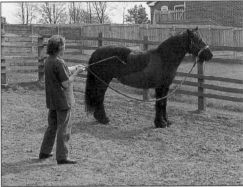

58, 59 (58) Horses on the lunge use sight (to gauge the trainer's body language) and hearing (to listen for vocal commands) to decide what their handler wants. Positioning yourself at the pony's hip and pointing the whip (if used) towards the hindquarters has the effect of sending him on. (59) Positioning yourself facing the forehand and pointing the whip towards the head is aimed at slowing down or stopping the pony. (NB: In both these photos of lunging, the rein used is a half-length lunging rein, which is easy to use and necessitates the trainer moving more with the horse or pony.)

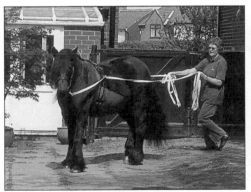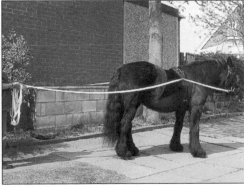

60, 61 Long reining. (60) Long reining offers more control than lunging, but the trainer needs to be quite fit and agile, even to keep up with a fast walking horse. Here, the long reins are fitted to the bit and passed through rings on a driving roller. Less skilled handlers should use a standard lunging cavesson and clip the reins to the side rings. (61) You can practise anywhere convenient. The horse listens for commands and can see your body position when you move from side to side to ask for changes of direction or specific movements. The reins are used to give a feel not only on the bit but also against the horse's sides to ask for movement away from their contact.

methods of loose schooling (**62**). It can also involve working with the horse on an ordinary lead rope, a double length lead rope (which is more convenient and safer as it gives you more controlled space should the horse become difficult), a controller head collar or halter of some kind, or a nose chain for extra control.

From the point of view of vision, it can be fun and good training working a horse over all sorts of objects on the ground, from various pole patterns and plastic sheets to obstacle courses made out of cones, upturned tubs or buckets, jump stands without the cups or any other safe equipment you can think of. The horse has to put his head down to see the items on the ground. He can see fairly clearly down his nose to graze and also, therefore, poles and other items that he has to negotiate. It is a wonderful way of getting the horse to look where he is going, to put his head down, which always has a relaxing effect on a horse and so enables him to concentrate and absorb lessons better, to listen to the trainer and watch where he is being taken and what he is being asked to do, and also to feel closer to the trainer as he/she is right next to him.

When your ground work takes place at a distance from the horse, as in lunging and loose schooling, the horse will watch your body position and movements (i.e. body language) minutely. He is superb at picking up your position, attitude and slightest movements, so you have to make sure that you get it right and are consistent. Horses communicate a good deal with each other by means of body positions and attitudes and easily transfer this innate skill to their connection with humans.

You can adopt a soft or submissive posture, by no means necessarily looking down away from the horse, but softly and in a welcoming way. The horse will sooner or later, according to how used he is to this sort of work, come to you calmly to be with you and maybe enquire what is coming next. If you so much as harden your gaze and stare at him, you will see that he notices this subtle change immediately and is instantly more on his guard. A more aggressive stance and actions, standing

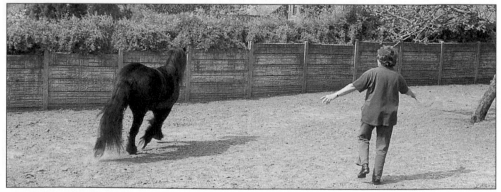

62 Horse and owner playing at loose 'schooling'. This can be great fun for pony and handler and many horses and owners find that it enhances their relationship and communication skills. Horses know very well that they cannot be caught and, depending on their mood and the attitude the handler is giving out, they may be very cooperative or enjoy second guessing what is coming next by watching their owner like a hawk (horses spot every tiny movement and change in posture) and deftly avoiding the issue as a game.

confidently, moving your arms in one or more directions, will send the horse away from you, but not necessarily in a frightened way; more playfully in my experience if he knows you well and understands the game.

Horses will also sometimes copy the movements of someone on the ground, without being asked and often when you are not expecting it. An old Thoroughbred I had, who was an angel under saddle but pretty dangerous on the ground, took amazingly well to doing ground work with me both on a lead and at liberty. He seemed really interested and watched me closely all the time to see what we were doing, copying my actions step for step, skidding to a halt next to me from a run both on a loose lead and at liberty, performing school patterns and really seeming to generally enjoy it all.

While teaching the Fell Pony and her owner to whom this book is dedicated, I demonstrated on foot the amount of crossing I wanted in shoulder-in. The pony started walking alongside me and adopted correct flexion and leg position next to me. The owner, who was riding her, and I were stunned, as we thought the pony was not even paying us any attention. The owner just sat there and the pony did shoulder-in alongside me for several steps. She actually lowered her head and looked at my feet and legs, obviously bringing them into the best view for her. She has done all this several times since, but we cannot seem to get her to do it for *travers*. In fact, she seems to tell us: 'No, you're flexing the wrong way. It's this way', and then does shoulder-in instead.

VISION AND RIDING

The easiest and most suitable job that a domesticated horse's eyesight best equips him for is relaxed hacking or riding with a fairly natural head carriage in open areas (where horses feel safest) (63), or drawing a vehicle under similar circumstances. Racing and endurance, at least as far as vision is concerned, are also suitable, because the head carriage is not restricted in these sports, and neither is it in some Western sports.

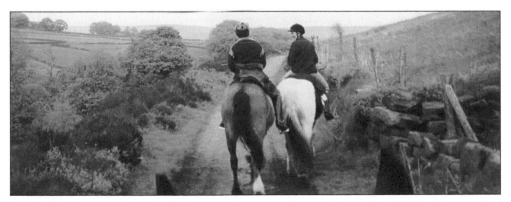

63 Hacking in open countryside mimics a horse's inclination to look far ahead in its natural environment and to travel around its area, and it often gives both horse and rider the chance to visit areas they would not normally see. Organized rides (not necessarily competitive) often take place over private land normally closed to the public. Most horses seem to feel at home in areas with wide views, probably because of their much more distant view of the world than ours.

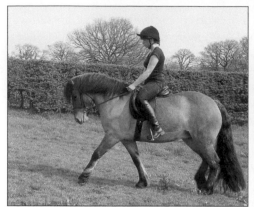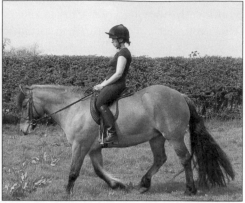

64, 65 (64) To the uninitiated, this overflexed posture of the head and neck might look attractive and correct, but this pony's forward vision is quite restricted, which is hardly a fair way to expect her to work. (65) This less demanding posture presents a happier picture and allows the pony a clearer view of her route.

Restricting the head carriage to a style and posture some people consider 'correct' or desirable (as described below) can effectively blind a horse (64, 65). This has been quite widely known for some years, yet still many people insist that horses must assume the posture known as 'on the bit', with the front of the face on or just a little in front of 'the vertical', an imaginary vertical line from the forehead down to the ground. More worryingly, the current fashion is for horses to be made to go, depending on their equestrian discipline, with their muzzles even behind this line, sometimes very much behind and even with the chin close to the chest. This ugly and counterproductive posture can be seen during schooling/training, exercising and competition.

It is no wonder that horses are reluctant to assume this posture naturally for more than a few seconds without a good deal of persuasion, cajoling and, sometimes, even coercion, because they cannot see ahead to where they are going or much to the side, either. Can you imagine having an opaque sunshade fixed very low in front of your eyes so that you can only see down to the ground for about a yard in front of your feet, and then being asked to run, sometimes quite fast, and jump obstacles in this state, at the same time having your head held or strapped down by the nose and by a metal bar in your mouth so that you cannot raise it to see where you are going? This is what many riders and trainers demand of their horses.

It is a common sight to see horses fighting to raise and tilt their heads when jumping so that they can actually see the obstacle at which, they know from experience, they are being aimed (66, 67). Their riders also may be fighting their struggling horse for control of speed and direction, which is why considerable force, often via strong (potentially painful) bits, is applied. The reason that horses do jump obstacles is probably that they have managed to see the obstacle on the approach some distance away and remember its height and structure as they get closer and it becomes less and less discernible. They finally jump it from memory.

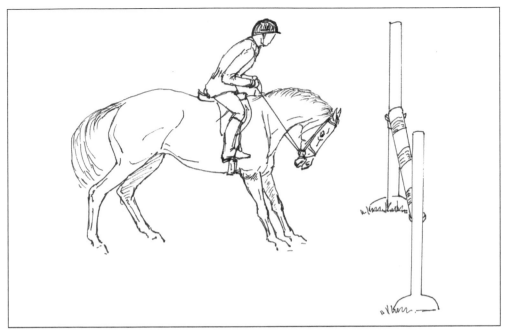

66 This horse is wisely putting on the brakes because he cannot see the jump. He could not jump well without much more freedom of his head and neck.

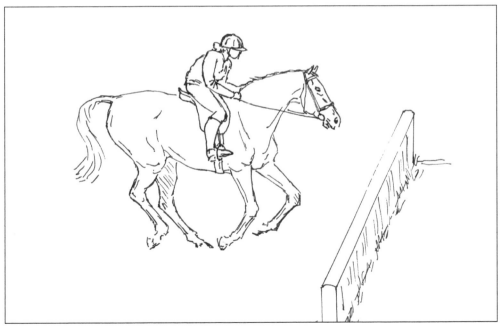

67 This horse's rider is letting him have a clear view of the jump she is asking him to tackle. With his head in this position he can bring the jump into clear view and judge his effort accurately.

If the rider is, indeed, fighting for control, it surely indicates that the horse is not yet well enough schooled/trained to be jumping at this level and is not habituated to responding to the rider's aids when fairly applied. Temperament plays a part and some horses hot up (become excited and hard to control) because of the physical activity of cantering or galloping and jumping, which gets the adrenaline going. Others may do so because of the apprehension of knowing what is going to happen and what is expected of them. Elite competition horses are normally selected on the basis of temperament as well as ability, and those who are just too hard to control may be rejected at this level, no matter how talented. As a top trainer once said: 'All the talent in the world is no good if you cannot control it'.

It is not only in jumping that we see horses being asked to perform with their heads in a restricted position. From my experience, observation and clear memory, this is happening more today than in previous decades. Horses working in various disciplines on the flat, at all levels, can be seen regularly being worked with their heads 'behind the vertical' and their necks stiff and shortened, often kinked down just in front of the withers. This, in turn, leads to a stiff back.

The reason the fashion has grown is because understanding of how a riding horse should go seems to have become gradually distorted in some quarters over the last couple of generations. People seem to have become 'front end orientated'. Getting the horse 'on the bit', which is supposed to mean comfortably accepting the bit and rounding his body lightly up to its tactful (definite, but light and empathetic) contact, has become a not so magnificent obsession, because instead of concentrating on the engagement and propulsive power of the hindquarters to achieve this state, many riders are now being urged and taught by instructors to 'get his head in' because it is felt that this 'frame', 'outline' or 'shape' is what the judges want to see. They also seem to believe that once the head is in, however this is achieved, it will automatically mean that the horse can go correctly in the rest of his body (68, 69). This is not so. It can lead to discomfort, pain, stiffness, resistance and a distressed, reluctant horse.

This fashion has led, I believe, to riders also becoming very dependent on their hands, as they use them constantly to position and hold in their horses' heads (with or without training aids or 'gadgets'), instead of relying on their seats for balance and security and allowing the horse freely to 'come through from behind', to use a fashionable term, without the energy being blocked in the forehand. Not everyone rides in this way, but so many do that it needs addressing.

Although this book is not a manual on the skills and principles of riding, a short explanation here will help to explain why the current fashion is, surely, unkind and unfair, because it must make horses uncomfortable and deprive them of the facility to see where they are going. From a safety viewpoint, it is also foolish. Naturally, horses who cannot see their track ahead must experience a level of psychological anxiety, if not fear, particularly when they know that obstacles are on that track. They can sometimes be seen to collide with objects, people and fences. Inability to see ahead also causes refusals at fences, run outs, poor jumping performance, rushing out of anxiety and lack of attention to the rider's aids. Falls in such circumstances are a not uncommon occurrence.

68 The rider is sitting back on her buttocks, bracing against the stirrups and applying a harsh contact on the bit. The horse has responded, this time, by flexing too far the other way in an effort to escape the action of the bit.

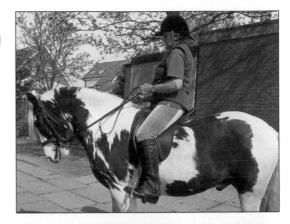

69 A badly positioned rider pulling on the rein causes the horse to resist the bit action by raising his head and pushing outwards with his jaw against its pressure. Horses often try to do this when their vision is restricted so that they can improve their view of their surroundings.

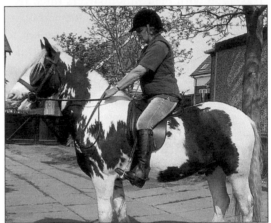

RIDING TO AIM FOR

Although a horse has four legs, the job of propulsion belongs mainly to the hind two. The front legs move the body on to a lesser extent. A healthy, reasonably athletically fit horse should be capable of carrying about a sixth of his own weight without undue stress, but even this load does affect his posture and way of going. The spine or vertebral column is made up of many variously shaped bones (vertebrae). These provide attachment for some muscles and provide a canal to house the spinal cord, an extension of the brain. The vertebrae articulate against each other and are cushioned by cartilaginous pads. The spine is not very flexible, except in the neck and tail region, but it can bend or flex laterally and longitudinally to a limited extent along most of its length. The lumbosacral joint, between the loin or lumbar vertebrae and the sacrum, is situated at the croup (the highest point of the hindquarters). The sacrum comprises five vertebrae fused together as one and so it is not at all flexible. Behind the sacrum are the caudal/tail vertebrae.

The central part of the vertebral column (the thoracic and lumbar sections) has a slight natural arch from the shoulders/withers to the croup (70, 71). This adds to its strength. The very heavy abdominal contents are slung underneath the thoracic and lumbar vertebrae from various soft tissues. The vertebral column is therefore bearing weight from below. When a rider mounts, the vertebral column is also bearing weight from above. If the horse can be trained to raise his back in order to emphasize his spinal arch (or 'vertebral bow', as it is often called) and so counteract the weight of the rider and saddle, this will help him to bear this weight with less effort and so lessen the chance of injury from stress and strain.

From a rider's point of view, horses are much more pleasant and manoeuvrable (and, therefore, safer) to ride if they are 'light in hand' (i.e. not leaning or boring down on the bit and creating firm, even heavy pressure on the rider's hands, but travelling with their hindquarters tilted from the lumbosacral joint, down, forward and under the body a little, inevitably bringing with them the hind legs). This 'tucking his bottom under' is equivalent to the famous pelvic tilt so familiar and essential to dancers, gymnasts and enthusiasts of yoga and Pilates. It strengthens the posture of the back in horses and humans and, in the former, makes weight

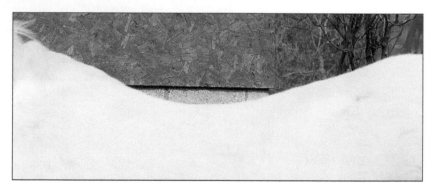

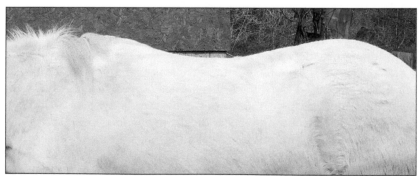

70, 71 (70) The natural line of a pony's back, which takes its shape from the dorsal processes of the spinal vertebrae. (71) The pony can clearly lift her back noticeably, flexing it longitudinally, as shown by the bottom of the wooden panel on the wall behind her.

72 A good head carriage. The horse's vision is not being restricted and the kind contact on the bit is acceptable to him. Via gentle pulses on one rein, the rider has asked him to 'give' to its pressure. In response, the horse has arched his neck a little, flexed at the poll (the atlanto-occipital joint or 'Yes joint') and his poll is, correctly, the highest point of his outline or posture, with his face just in front of the vertical. He has slightly opened his mouth to accept and gently play with his bit. The joints involved in this latter movement are those just below the ears between the lower jaw or mandible and the skull, the temporomandibular joints or 'jaw joints'.

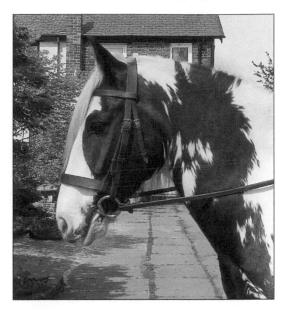

carrying easier. Opinions still vary on whether or not 'tucking his bottom under' actually causes the horse to move his centre of balance backwards a little, but, when done properly, it does have the effect of making the horse better balanced, more agile and better able to comply with the rider's aids. The horse is going more from the 'back end' and pushing forwards strongly, using his forehand less to 'haul' himself along and feeling lighter in hand, partly because of good posture and balance and partly because the rider is not forcing the head in. A good, educated rider will use his or her legs and a light seat to activate the hind legs and quarters, encouraging the horse to 'lift' his forehand and stretch and arch his head and neck out and forwards and maybe up, depending on the horse's stage of development.

So what about 'on the bit'? There is no doubt that horses can go as described both at liberty and with a rider without any contact at all on the bit. However, initially, it helps them to balance under weight if there is a tactful guiding contact with the bit (72). The outside rein is the 'master' rein, which guides and supports the horse as far as balance, speed and direction are concerned. Contact via the outside rein with the bit/mouth should usually be about the same as you would use to hold a young child's hand to guide him across the road; firm enough to control him but light enough to feel reassuring, and not gripping uncomfortably. Depending on the horse, the contact is variable, but it should never cause distress or pain. To indicate direction left or right, the outside rein is pressed sideways against the horse's neck just in front of the withers, which turns the horse in much better balance, and more lightly, than pulling him round with the inside rein. The inside rein is used lightly and intermittently to ask for 'give'

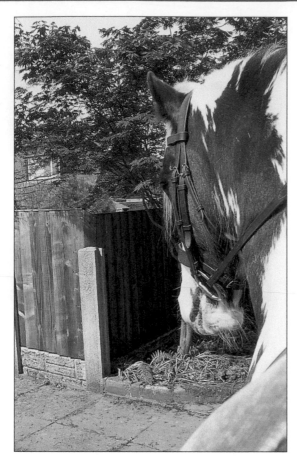

73 Correct, slight flexion for turns and circles. The rider should just be able to see the corner of the horse's inside eye and the rim of his nostril.

in the jaw at the temporomandibular joints just below the ear (the noseband must be loose enough to permit this) and to ask for flexion/bend to the inside of a turn or circle at the atlanto-axial joint, or 'No' joint (73).

With this way of going and these more effective and lighter aids (accompanied by seat and leg aids and positioning), the horse can perform accurately, willingly and lightly, and will hold his head in a suitable position for him to have full use of his eyesight. Surprisingly to some, this is often just in front of the vertical (the correct standard), without any 'holding in' or force.

Riding technique and ethics comprise a big subject that is really outside the scope of this book. However, I do feel that, in the interests of equine welfare and in the light of our current, scientifically proven knowledge of equine physiology and vision, much more effort will have to be made to see that this knowledge is widely disseminated within all levels of the horse world, so that it has beneficial practical effects on how horses are schooled, managed and ridden. Administrative bodies and teaching organisations need to ensure that any regulations they lay down in this regard are actually implemented in practice (i.e. in training, competition and examinations), penalties being applied to riders who fail to act in accordance with them.

SHYING AND 'SPOOKING'

Because horses' vision is geared to detecting movement and recognizing shape rather than to discerning objects in clear, sharp detail, they often tend to shy or spook because they cannot identify items as humans can. Anything that is moved from its usual place constitutes a change in the area and this, to the horse, can mean danger. Objects appearing where they are not usually found seem to be more threatening than those that are simply removed. The horse's instinct sees such an object as a possible predator and he may stop dead in his tracks, snorting to try to smell for any clues, ears pricked hard forward to listen for any helpful sounds and moving his head around to try to assess what it is. He may leap sideways or he may take to his heels to get away from the object. Another manoeuvre is to face the object (**74**). The horse performs what amounts almost to a turn about the forehand as he fixes his gaze on the object to keep it in view and swivels his hindquarters sideways around it, after which he may straighten up and proceed, snorting and prancing, with his attention focused backwards to check that it is not following him.

Some riders find this sort of behaviour quite funny, but it really scares others. However, it is not a safe way for a horse to behave. When being driven, it can be even more dangerous, as the horse may play up to the extent that the vehicle is overturned and its occupants thrown out. Driving horses often wear blinkers to restrict their view to the side and behind, thus giving them less to fuss about, but this does not stop horses reacting to things they are approaching. In these cases, encouragement from the driver may not be enough. He or she may need to get down from the vehicle and lead the horse past, or have another person do so. Because these reactions are natural and quite common among some horses, ways of dealing with shying need to be considered.

74 This pony is concerned about the lawn mower and has tilted her head to bring it more clearly into focus with her right eye. Ideally, the rider would halt and let the pony investigate it, but this may not be possible where there are pedestrians or traffic. If the pony continued in this vein, she could end up swinging her quarters well to the left as she tried to keep the mower in view. The rider is not helping by turning her body towards the object and looking at it.

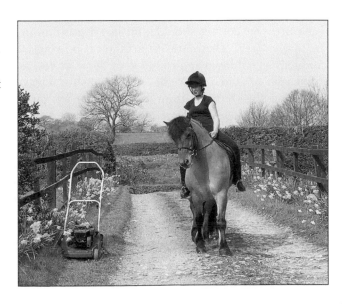

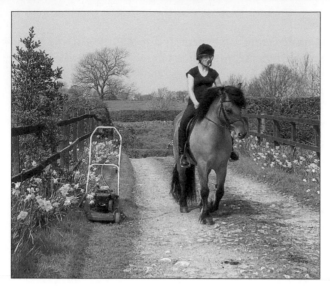

75 Well corrected. This is how to tackle this sort of situation, by flexing the pony away from a frightening object (in 'head-away' or shoulder-in), looking ahead to where you want to go, and giving firm aids to walk on. The pony can still see the mower, but her body is under control, her quarters will not swing out and she will pass under her rider's direction rather than skittering past in a less safe manner.

Ideally, from an education viewpoint, you want the horse to be able to go up to the object, have a good look and smell, possibly touch it with his muzzle and even a forefoot and generally satisfy himself that it poses no threat. This is fine if you are in an area where it is safe to do this. However, if you are in traffic or a crowded place, or the horse has spooked at this object before, you need to get him to go past it under control. It is worth noting that horses often shy in the same place and going in the same direction as they have done before, even if the original cause of the shy has gone. This is because they form habits very easily.

The way to get a horse to go past a threatening object under control is to put him into shoulder-in, or 'head away' as it is sometimes called (75). This does not have to be a dressage correct shoulder-in, just a position in which the horse is flexed away from the object. Therefore, if the object is on your left, sit upright and drop your seat and legs as far down and round your horse as you can. Flex him to the right with the right rein around your right leg and push sideways with the left rein to move his forehand slightly away from it. Point your left hip up the route you wish to follow, press weight down into your left heel and stirrup and look where you want to go. Your right leg taps and pushes intermittently on his side to get him moving. You are in control of the situation and the horse knows it.

This technique does not prevent the horse seeing the object, which he can do towards his rear out of his left eye for some steps (although it will 'disappear' eventually), but it does put him physically in a flexed position in which his body is under reasonable control. Maintain a calm, firm attitude and use confident vocal aids such as 'walk on'. Do not praise him, by saying 'good boy' or anything similar, until he has in fact been good by passing the object despite his fear. Then praise him by stroking (not patting) his lower neck and using your voice in a pleased tone.

CARE AND MANAGEMENT

Horses usually seem to prefer a stable with a view out over the surrounding area (76). This is not surprising, as they are animals of the wide open spaces, long-sighted and with a need, in nature, to scan their environment for predators. It is noticeable that horses turned out in paddocks with rising ground or hillocks very frequently stand on the highest areas, just resting, socializing and looking around.

If you have a choice, it seems appropriate to choose a stable in an area that will allow your horse to look around rather than stand staring at a close-up, dull view (77). Again, most horses enjoy having two or more viewing outlets in their stables. These can be closed off to wind and rain, when strictly necessary (as horses always prefer to put their heads out), by having the doors to their outlets made of some kind of transparent but unbreakable material, and still giving the horses a view out.

Have a good look around your yard in relation to the view. Windbreaks are a boon in some locations, but assess the whole site and see where man-made or natural obstructions to the view could be taken down, modified or moved to open up more of a vista for the horses.

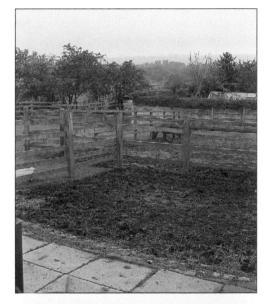

76 The view from this stable allows the occupant a view for miles around, which certainly seems to be appreciated.

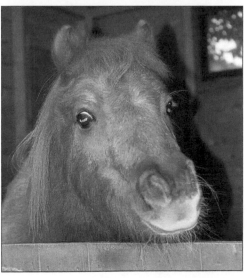

77 Small ponies often have an unhappy and stressful time when stabled simply because the doors of their stables are too high for them to see over without craning their necks (and potentially straining both their necks and backs) or trying to stand on the cross-members of their stable doors. I have known more than one pony jump up like a dog and hook their forelegs over the door just so that they could see the outside world, something their owners thought amusing, but causes stress and strain to the pony's back. This stable, however, has a door specially made for the pony's height, so he is quite content.

PHOTOPERIODICITY OR THE EFFECTS OF LIGHT

Like all creatures that do not live in total darkness, the horse's annual cycle of life and breeding and his daily one of activity, eating, drinking and resting are governed by light. As mentioned earlier, horses are most active around dawn and dusk when the light is dim and they can see best (**78**). They are quieter and stiller on dark nights and more active on moonlit ones. Bright light such as strong sunlight makes vision difficult for horses and, at liberty, they often rest more at such times.

In my opinion the new year starts at the winter solstice (December 21st in the northern hemisphere), the shortest day of the year, as this is when the natural year turns and the days start to lengthen again. Spring is on the way! As light enters the eyes through the pupils for a longer and longer period each day, the brain perceives this and signals changes in the hormones that are constantly being produced and circulated around the horses' bodies. Males and females must now be prepared for the breeding season in order to procreate their species. Although colts and stallions are stimulated by increasing light levels to produce the male hormone testosterone, the more complex cycle is that of the mare.

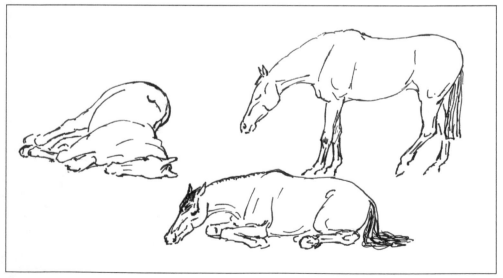

78 While some horses sleep or doze and others graze, at least one will be awake and alert to possible danger in the surrounding area. Horses seem to be most active in moderate light conditions around dawn and dusk.

Light enters the eye through the pupil and a message is passed along the optic nerve to the brain. This results in the pineal body (a small gland in the diencephalon or upper brain responsible for secreting a hormone called melatonin, which depresses sexual interest) reducing production of melatonin according to the increasing amount of light sensed. The horses respond by gradually feeling more and more like breeding. Part of the upper brain (the hypothalamus) senses the reduced levels of melatonin. In entire males of pubertal age and beyond, this ultimately results, via several steps, in increased production of testosterone in the testes. Testosterone is the male hormone that produces stallion-like tendencies. Interestingly, about three-quarters of geldings retain significant stallion characteristics, some more than others, so spring fever affects them as well as their entire colleagues.

The Oestrus Cycle (see also pp. 18, 19)

The reduced level of melatonin causes the hypothalamus to produce gonadotropin-releasing hormone (GnRH), which itself stimulates the pituitary gland in the diencephalon or upper brain in mares and pubertal fillies to produce follicle-stimulating hormone (FSH). This stimulates the ripening of follicles (fluid-filled sacs that develop around eggs in the ovaries of mares), which, as they grow, produce the hormone oestrogen. It is this hormone that causes mares to show the normal behavioural signs of being in season and which causes owners who do not understand or are not interested in breeding horses to complain that their mares are 'mare-ish' (!) or 'stroppy'. Mares are in season or oestrus for four or five days, being most fertile towards the end of that time, but in the early part of the breeding season their seasons are usually erratic and infertile.

Oestrogen has a negative feedback effect on the pituitary gland, which consequently reduces the production of FSH. The pituitary gland is also stimulated by oestrogen to produce luteinising hormone (LH), which causes the follicle to rupture and reduces oestrogen levels. The follicle releases the egg (called ovulation) into the Fallopian tube running from the ovary to the uterus, where it is available to be fertilized by one of the many sperm produced by a stallion at mating, should this occur. A blood clot (the corpus haemorrhagicum) forms in the space formerly occupied by the egg, and LH causes specialized luteal cells to invade the clot and change it into the corpus luteum, or yellow body. As this grows, it produces progesterone, the hormone that causes the mare to go out of season or enter the dioestrus part of her cycle, which lasts about 16 days. (The term used for the mare's usual state in winter, when most do not come into season at all, is anoestrus.)

As the progesterone level continues to rise and the oestrogen level to fall, another negative feedback effect occurs in the pituitary gland, triggering reduced production of LH and increased production of FSH. The uterus now produces yet another hormone, prostaglandin, to 'kill off' the yellow body in the ovary and stop it producing progesterone; this is necessary because progesterone inhibits the in-oestrus stage of the cycle. The hypothalamus detects the lower levels of progesterone and produces GnRH again, which stimulates production of FSH, and so the cycle repeats itself. Typically, oestrus lasts for five days and dioestrus for 16 days once the mare is cycling regularly in spring and summer.

There is some anecdotal evidence that horses kept in indoor stabling or free in indoor barns are not so quickly affected by light rays passing into the eye. This may be because they are not exposed to as much natural daylight and most such accommodation for horses is not equipped with full-spectrum light fittings equivalent to daylight. This topic is dealt with later in this section.

The Annual Cycle of Activity

Light affects all horses, even though some may not be able to respond to it like free ones. The effects of light on naturally living horses in the northern hemisphere are reviewed below.

By about February, despite it still being mid-winter as far as temperature and natural food availability are concerned, both mares and stallions (and, in domestic conditions, even geldings) are showing signs of 'silly' behaviour (i.e. restlessness, snorting, playing and squealing). Their winter coat is beginning to cast (moult) and mares start coming into season, albeit infertile ones, a fact noted by colts and stallions. About this time, stallions start becoming unfriendly towards sexually mature colts and the latter may leave, or be required to leave, the herd.

By the spring or vernal equinox, when the hours of darkness and daylight are equal, mares will be cycling more or less regularly and it only takes the growth of spring grass to cause them to start ovulating and, therefore, produce fertile seasons, which cause them to become truly interested in the stallion. Foaling in nature takes place in spring and summer (not mid-winter as it is often forced to do in domesticity) when the grass is at its most nutritious. Mares will come into season again and ovulate shortly after foaling and, at this so-called foal heat, they may well mate, though not always.

When the summer solstice occurs (about June 21st in the northern hemisphere, the longest day of the year), foals will probably be getting as much nourishment from the grass as from their dam's milk and they will start taking less and less milk. The dam may be pregnant again, but with good food and reducing demand for milk she can easily cope with both her foal and her fetus. By the time the fetus is at its most demanding, during the last three months of her pregnancy, the foal will be taking very little milk and natural weaning takes place at the time nature knows best, being nothing like the psychologically damaging process for mare and foal that it can be in domesticity, when foals are weaned early, at six months of age commonly, which is by no means normal for the species.

The autumn equinox, which, like the spring equinox, produces days and nights of about equal length, occurs on September 21st. Before this, given reasonable rainfall to promote grass growth, there will probably have been an 'autumn flush' of grass and other herbage. This enables the natural herd to put on some weight and store energy ready for the hard winter to come. Their interest in breeding is much reduced now. The mare's gestation or pregnancy period is about eleven months, and there is no point in having a foal born into natural conditions in late summer or early autumn, as it will not be sufficiently developed and independent to make it through the winter. The autumn growth of grass does not contain as much essential protein for growth as the spring growth.

The horses' yearly cycle is now coming full circle and, as the winter solstice approaches again, the reducing light levels will have reduced the hormones responsible for interest in breeding. The lower light level also puts the horses into 'saving' mode, as they preserve energy for keeping warm by being less active, which also allows them to use what food they can find to live off. By spring, they will be lean from meagre rations and some will not have made it through the long, dark, cold winter. The strongest and fittest (most suitable) for the conditions in which the herd finds itself will survive to procreate more of their type and, as the days lengthen after the winter solstice, the yearly cycle starts all over again.

Manipulating the Yearly Cycle

Some owners are very interested in manipulating their horses' natural cycles for their own ends; for example, those producing breeds such as flat-race Thoroughbreds and some other breeds that have their official birthdays on January 1st in the northern hemisphere (or some time during the summer in some southern hemisphere countries). This date was chosen when two-year-old racing became popular in the 18th and 19th centuries, so owners could get their youngsters onto the racecourse, looking well-grown and trained, earlier in the year. Breeders of some other breeds, for showing and competition, also want mature looking youngsters earlier in the season so that they have more chance of winning, or being sold. Various ruses have been devised to bring nature's system forward so that breeding and foaling start in what is often mid-winter, which is a completely unnatural time.

Bringing horses into show and breeding condition is controlled mainly by lengthening hours of daylight and, but only to a lesser extent, warmth and feeding. Many breeders put a great deal of clothing on their animals to try and trick their brains into believing that spring has arrived. They are attempting to cause early casting of the winter coat so that the horse or pony will carry a short, glossy summer coat much earlier than natural in the season. This must be really unpleasant and rather distressing for the horse or pony, no matter how well the rugs fit. It is more effective, and cheaper, particularly as electric lighting is relatively cheap compared with heating and buying expensive rugs for each animal, to increase the horse's exposure to increasing hours of full-spectrum light, which his brain will pick up as lengthening days. Excessive feeding and rugging up are not good for horses, so feed should be increased only in moderation, and clothing likewise. The way to use light to control horses' natural cycles (stallions, mares and geldings) is as follows:

• To encourage summer condition, from the winter solstice start exposing your horses or ponies to 16 hours a day of full-spectrum light, both natural and artificial. If your animals are in indoor stabling complexes, make sure that they have as much outdoor time as is reasonably possible, wearing appropriate rugs. By all means increase the feeding carefully and keep the horses cosily warm, but certainly not muffled up and overloaded with rugs. Light is the crucial factor and it also produces a better summer-type coat than when just rugs and feed are relied upon. Studs selling foals and yearlings in late summer and autumn, and aiming at keeping their summer condition until the sales, can start this regime gradually after the summer solstice, the idea being that the horses' brains do not sense a reduction in daylight entering the eyes.

- Buy some full-spectrum light strips or bulbs to simulate natural, full-spectrum daylight (called white light). However, even though it says on the packaging that the strip or bulb emits 'white light', it may not actually be full-spectrum. It may be simply that the strip or bulb is white in colour, and this will not produce what you are looking for. In the UK, successful strips and bulbs have been used from the Daystar and Activa brands. Hospitals used to treating people with seasonal affective disorder (SAD), or 'winter blues', use panels for varying lengths of time. You should be able to acquire this equipment through any good electrical shop. Ordinary candescent light bulbs work if they are at least 100 watts, and preferably twice that much. However, cheap blue-spectrum fluorescent strips should not be bought, as these not only do not seem to work at all, but are believed to cause headaches and depression in humans and, maybe, in other animals, who may show irritable behaviour and lethargy when exposed to them for long periods. I believe that it is the rapid flicker of these blue-spectrum tubes that is at least partly responsible for the problem.
- If the horses are exposed to daylight (i.e. not indoors) during the day, you can count the hours between dawn and dusk and put on your lights morning and/or evening to make up a total of 16 hours daily of full-spectrum light. For this technique to work, it appears that the horses must be exposed to eight hours of darkness. Interestingly, it was found some years ago that just one hour's exposure to light between 2am and 3am has the same effect, but you would need a timer switch to use this method. A dimmer switch would also be helpful, as it is very unpleasant to have a bright light suddenly switched on in the middle of the night.
- Animals required to breed early in the spring or late winter can have hormonal treatment from your veterinary surgeon, as well as being kept warm (not in a stuffy, hot environment) and having their diets gradually and carefully increased, but the main and most practical way of achieving your aim is the increase in light exposure.

Light may well be able to be used as therapy, as in humans, although I have no experience of this and have not heard of it being carried out in horses. If you have a horse who seems fractious during the short, dark days, it is well worth discussing it with your veterinary surgeon. There are many reasons for 'unwanted' behaviour in horses, but the important aspect is not so much that the people dealing with the horse find it a problem, but that the horse is obviously not particularly happy. Excess feeding of starch, insufficient feeding of fibre, uncomfortable clothing, being genuinely cold or too hot, lack of attention to clean water and adequate clean, dry bedding, freedom and company are all reasons for behavioural difficulties in horses. Attention should be given to the whole management system as far as it affects that particular horse, but increased full-spectrum light may well play a part in his improvement.

COLOUR THERAPY

It can be tricky to recommend conventional colour therapy for horses, as they appear not to be able to see all the colours seen by humans, although there is still research work going on in this field. Some owners are convinced that their horses can distinguish yellow and green. This is from both general experience and their own experiments, although the horses may not see these colours as humans do.

Most stables are not painted in colours aimed at affecting a horse's mental attitudes to life. Some stables are so dark and dingy that it seems they must be really depressing despite the fact that horses prefer dim light to darkness or bright light. I used to visit a yard in which the stables were painted pale blue above the kicking boards and the kicking boards themselves were green. The owner said that these colours best mimicked what the horse would see when out – a blue sky above green grass, which seems logical – although the bedding was always lovely, shiny, golden straw.

In humans, colours are known to have definite effects on psychologically disturbed people. Red can make people angry; orange can liven us up and stimulate us to action; pink is said to make us feel warm, romantic and happy; yellow is said to promote brain activity and so is good for studies and classrooms; green is healing and calming and blue is relaxing (and apparently both colours make us feel generous and like buying things!); lilac is cooling and restful; and purple is said to be a very magical, spiritual colour.

It would be interesting to try altering the colours of a horse's stable to see what, if any, effects that seemed to have. Would a bad-tempered mare be any sweeter if her stable was pink, and would a hyperactive stallion calm down if his box was blue or purple?

Many horses are known not to like walking on the colour black; they seem to see it as a hole, which is useful to know because many horsebox ramps are black and loading problems are now very common in the horse world, although for other reasons as well. When black is changed for green or red, it is found that many horses load up the ramp much easier.

The reflection of light on water, making a moving carpet of bright, shiny silver, can be extremely startling to some horses, not always young ones. I have kept and ridden horses near the sea for many years and am used to their reactions to this effect when first taken onto a beach. However, I didn't expect anything much from my very worldy-wise 24-year-old Thoroughbred mare on visiting the seashore after a change of yards. The tide was right out on the flat expanse of wet sand and had left the usual ripple shapes with their little 'valleys' filled with water. The mare had clearly never been on a beach in her long life or seen such a glittering, shifting carpet of light spread out for miles before her. We had a very close and trusting relationship, but it still took me about ten minutes of patient cajoling to get her to descend the slope to the beach, snorting and back-pedalling all the way down. At the bottom the sea had left a shallow pool of water which, in any other environment, she would have paddled through without thinking, having no concerns about water, but which here presented a huge challenge because of the bright light reflecting off it. I let her take her time. She eventually called on her considerable reserves of courage, her perception and assessment of the situation and her well-practised ability to make decisions that suited both herself and her rider.

Using all her senses, except taste, she judged the circumstances carefully, despite trembling like a leaf. She had a tremendous leap, but knew that I did not want her to jump the pool, so she tested the water with one hoof, smelled it (being salty it did not smell like any other water she had ever come across), dropped and tipped her head to one side to get a closer look and then gingerly, lifting her feet very high, tiptoed all around the edge of the pool. This, of course, landed her among dazzling rivulets of water as far as the eye could see. She stood snorting and trembling, looking all around, then started to do a natural piaffe. At a hint from me, she went forward and passaged for about half a mile along the beach; then we turned, my heart in my mouth in case she bolted for the slope. The sun was now in our eyes, which I now know must have made things even worse for her, but she just maintained her passage. I took her past the end of the slope and she actually began to walk loftily as we turned again, splashed through the pool at the bottom of the slope and marched up it, giving a massive sigh of relief at the top. What a horse!

Chapter 12
THE SENSE OF TOUCH

Because nearly everything we do with horses involves touching them, it is surprising how little attention the sense of touch receives and how much it is, sometimes inadvertently or unknowingly, abused. Unlike their sense of vision, horses' sense of touch is very much like ours, although many people think that their pain threshold is lower than ours in general, which makes it even more important to treat them with consideration. The big difference is that the main way horses investigate objects is not by touching them with their fingers and hands, because they do not have any (although they may use their forefeet as part of the investigation process), but by using their muzzles.

The muzzle is used for smell, touch and taste and is extremely important to the horse as a way of gathering information. This is one reason why the area should be treated with much greater respect and sensitivity than it often is. It is well known how sensitive human mouths are (both the lips and the insides of the mouth, where the tiniest sore spot can be quite painful), yet some riders abuse their horse's mouth in such a way that they must think a horse's ability to feel in this area is nothing like ours; in fact, it is just the same (79).

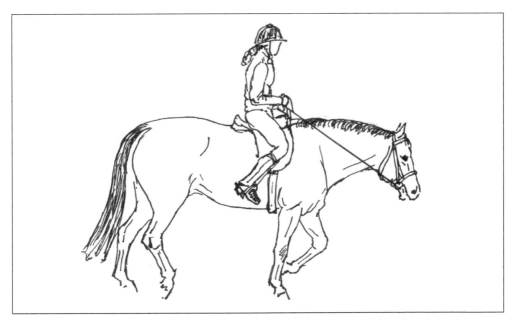

79 A horse's responses to touch can easily be dulled by this kind of riding. This horse is leaning on the bit and, therefore, on the forehand, with his balance too far forward. The rider is spurring the horse's sides to try and improve the situation.

Other areas that are very sensitive are the withers, the girth area and the flanks or sides. Many horses, particularly green ones, are very touchy around the area between their hind legs, where the genitals or mammary glands are sited, in the groin area, underneath their tails and, often, generally about the head. Although the feet themselves are comparatively insensitive, many horses do not like their heels, feet and lower legs being handled, and few will permit it without specific handling and training. All this should be taught on the stud before the foal leaves his dam, along with general good behaviour when led. This is good initial training for a youngster on the way to becoming a well-mannered riding horse. Naturally, the horse himself may have a very different view of all this but, unfortunately for him, in our society and culture he is rarely allowed much choice as to whether or not he works or who handles and works with him.

Some horses seem to be naturally welcoming of humans and the strange things they do to them, whereas others, regardless of training and perhaps because of poor or bad treatment in the past (weak or abusive), make it very clear that certain people are not welcome in their vicinity.

It was explained in chapter 1 how constant overstimulation of the nerve endings can cause lasting and sometimes permanent lack of response, resulting in hard-mouthed and dead-sided horses. Riding school animals are mainly subjected to beginner and novice riders. Unwittingly, such riders can ruin the horses' and ponies' responses because of their lack of skill. Other horses, perhaps surprisingly, can also be affected. Even some high-level competition horses, which you would expect to be sensitive and well-schooled, can be found, when passed down the market after retirement, to be quite insensitive to the aids because of the way they have been ridden. I have ridden and schooled horses from several different disciplines that have been dead to the leg, heavy in hand and poorly balanced (not always all in the same horse) because of the riding techniques used by their supposedly skilled competitive riders; not the best route to success, and certainly not pleasant for either horse or rider.

Horses that are allowed to use their free will regarding which horses, people and other animals may touch them are often quite protective of their own bodies, just as humans are. Horses in general seem to have an invisible limit around their bodies of varying distances. In a herd situation, only 'preferred associates' or favoured family members and friends are allowed voluntarily close enough to touch. Horses who are emotionally close to each other can be seen grazing together, very close physically (80) and often touching, particularly at the shoulders. Feral equids can be seen to start running from predators 25 metres or more away, whereas they will tolerate a non-preferred but non-aggressive associate up to about six metres away.

Some of the above matters in relation to management, handling and work are discussed below.

VIBRISSAE/WHISKERS

In common with many other animals, the horse has special 'feeler' hairs on his head, around the muzzle and eyes. However, whereas in other animals (e.g. cats, rabbits, pet mice and rats) these whiskers are often a source of pride to their owners, and maybe to the animals judging by the length of time they spend grooming them, in horses many owners are only too ready to clip them off for the sake of neatness. By doing this, the owner is depriving the horse of one of his most important items of sensory equipment.

Whiskers are not ordinary hairs. They seem particularly sensitive and specific in the messages they send to the brain. The vibrissae help horses to detect the presence of items, including food, on the ground in front of them and they can be seen to touch things with them before making closer contact with lips or nostrils. The ones around the eyes help horses in unnatural conditions such as transport, and also in very dark conditions, presumably to tell them when objects are near their heads so they can avoid knocking them.

Clipping the vibrissae off for the sake of so-called neatness is surely most unfair, and a change in attitude is long overdue in those horse people who approve of and do this. The argument that horses soon get used to being without them, and that these people have never noticed any adverse effects due to their lack, does not hold water. In Germany it has been unlawful for several years to clip off the vibrissae in view of their sensory importance, and some administrative organisations in the horse world are banning their removal. Congratulations to them for setting an example that I think all the others should follow.

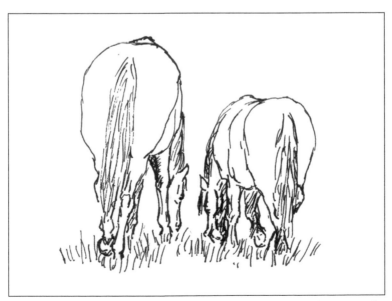

80 Good friends or close family members may graze very close to each other, often gently touching each other's bodies.

MUTUAL GROOMING

One of the most enjoyable things horses do with each other is perform mutual grooming. They stand head to tail and use their incisors (front teeth) and muzzles to rub, nuzzle and sometimes gently nip each other along the upper part of the neck, the withers and just behind the withers (mainly), and sometimes further along the upper part of the back and hindquarters (81). They stand with their ears flopped sideways or loosely back and often with their eyes half closed, looking anywhere from relaxed to ecstatic, and they do this for many minutes at a time. Some horses also try to do this with their owners. However, many owners, who have more traditional (hidebound?) views of the horse/human relationship, prevent mutual grooming and certainly do not return the favour, which is probably rather hurtful to the horse – a form of rejection from someone prominent in his life.

Mutual grooming is possibly the equivalent in horses to what a relaxing and pleasurable massage is to humans. They seem to use a fair amount of pressure when they do it, but never hurt each other. Usually, one horse will approach and offer to

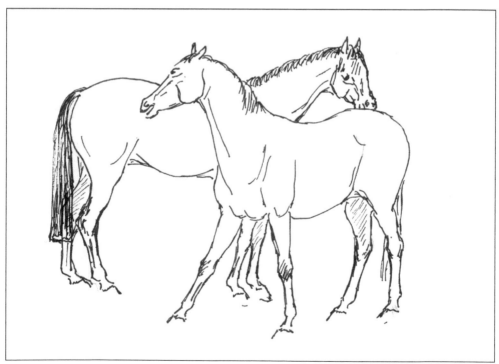

81 The practice known as mutual grooming is very popular between friends and, some believe, it is a getting-to-know-you activity, establishing positions and bonds. Studies have shown that it lowers the heart rate and relaxes horses. They nuzzle each other quite firmly with their lips and they scrape with their incisor teeth, the area receiving most attention being around the withers and part way along the back. As this is an important equine social activity, it is important that horses are not kept isolated from others and are allowed the chance to perform mutual grooming.

groom and then the other will return the favour. I have seen free stallions mutual groom with their offspring, even with young foals who were not able to reach up to the normal areas to take part, but groomed their sire further down his side. Friends often mutually groom, and mares do it with their offspring and other herd members. An interesting example is when my dog accepts it quite happily from a friend's Shetland Pony, which she has done several times but, of course, has no idea that she is expected to perform it back. The pony nuzzles the dog's head as well as her shoulders and back, and the dog clearly pushes back against him. The owner feels that her pony is delighted that he has found someone small enough for him to groom.

Mutual grooming certainly seems to be a form of bonding or of cementing a good relationship, but it can also be used when horses are getting to know each other quite well. When two friends have not been free together for some time, they may often be seen to mutual groom for quite a while on first being turned out together, even before settling to graze.

There does not seem to be any kind of hierarchical jockeying for position in mutual grooming. 'Highs' and 'lows' alike in the heirarchy seem to mutual groom if they basically get on with each other but, according to my own observations, it is noticeable that flies in the ointment (i.e. field bullies) do not seem to be able to acquire mutual grooming partners.

Some horses try to rub their heads on their riders when their bridles are removed after work, particularly if they have been hot and sweaty. This is obviously meant to deal with itching after work, but many people take it as a sign of lack of respect and that the horse regards them as inferior in status to him. I think this is very unlikely. Surely, if this were so, there would be other signs of the horse trying to get the upper hand. Personally, I do not mind if a horse I am very friendly with rubs his head on me. With a horse I do not know well, or who is 'pushy', I usually remove the bridle and then firmly rub and scratch where the bridle has been (if the horse wants me to) rather than letting him rub his head on me.

When I remove the saddle I usually give a horse a good, firm scratch and rub in the saddle and girth areas and, although the girth area in particular is very sensitive, horses really love this little service. Their top lips pout and quiver, their heads go up and their ears back. When I stop they often ask for more by pointing with their muzzles to the areas that need a bit more attention.

Mutual grooming is known to cause a drop in a horse's heart rate and be very relaxing, although I do not know if any work has been done to find out if it also reduces levels of blood cortisol (the 'stress hormone'). It would be interesting to know. Probably, bodywork therapies such as hand rubbing and massage, careful body brushing and wisping have a similar effect. I am an equine shiatsu therapist and I know from their reactions that horses most definitely love this therapy once they experience it and understand it, and they show every sign of being deeply relaxed. It has lasting effects as well. More information about hand rubbing, massage and shiatsu can be found later in this chapter (see Therapies).

Some years ago I saw a television programme featuring a farmer who had installed large, stiff, electrically-operated rotary brushes in his milking parlours, which his cows queued up to use before and after milking. The cows could use the brushes or not, as they wished. Some hogged them and had to be moved on because they were causing a cow jam. Apparently, milk yields had risen noticeably and the cows were quieter and more content – all because of a good scrub from the brushes. This seems like a good idea for horses, except that their long manes could become caught up in them.

HOUSING FOR HORSES

The traditional idea that horses should not be allowed to touch each other in stables is still rife throughout many quarters of the horse world. This is highly unnatural and, where friends are concerned, not conducive to their well-being as it causes them distress. Single 'cells' in which horses are confined most of the time and from which they can only look out at other horses without being able to touch, smell, taste or keep any kind of normal, social company do not in any way satisfy the emotional requirements of horses. Many people have the firmly ingrained idea that this kind of housing is 'safest' for their horses, who will, they believe, regularly injure and upset each other and even themselves if allowed contact. Stables like this are only one step better than solitary confinement, a situation which deeply distresses most horses and ponies. Because horses clearly derive so much enjoyment, reassurance, pleasure and comfort from being able physically to touch each other, surely we should be criticizing and rejecting this type of accommodation and recommending and demanding more appropriate designs in the interests of equine welfare and well-being (82).

Horses kept in communal situations (e.g. corrals, yards at least part of which are covered, indoor pens large enough for two or more horses or ponies), or those kept out at least part of the time with access to shelters, run-in sheds, open barns and the like, are, to the sensitive and observant, clearly calmer and more content and fulfilled than those kept mainly apart from other horses in single-stable accommodation. The usual excuse that horses able to touch each other significantly (not merely sniff each other through grilled 'chat holes' in the walls) tend to fight, tear each other's rugs and try to get over their dividing partitions may be true in cases where non-preferred associates (enemies or those who just do not get on) are stabled next to each other. This is bad horse management and needs to be avoided. In free conditions, such horses would tend to avoid each other. In feral situations they would probably not even stay in the same herd for long; therefore, in domestic situations they should certainly not be forced to live and work near each other.

Some people refuse to allow friends to be stabled next to each other, even when they cannot touch, because, it is claimed, they form an 'impossible bond'; that is, they become distressed when separated for work or other reasons. In my wide experience this only happens when the horses concerned have an insufficiently strong relationship with their human associates, and it is usually due to weakness or aggressiveness of character and actions on the part of those humans. Horse handlers need to inspire trust in their equine charges and to be always calm, firm and positive in all their dealings with them. (A period working or training in any decent professional yard will teach these qualities – or confirm that the person concerned is not cut out for coping with horses.)

The two golden rules for single-stable accommodation as far as horse-to-horse relationships are concerned are (1) only friendly horses should be stabled next to, or even near, each other; and (2) horses should be allowed to nuzzle each other over their dividing partitions by having at least part of them at the height of the horses' withers. The remaining section can be higher where the main feeding station is sited, although

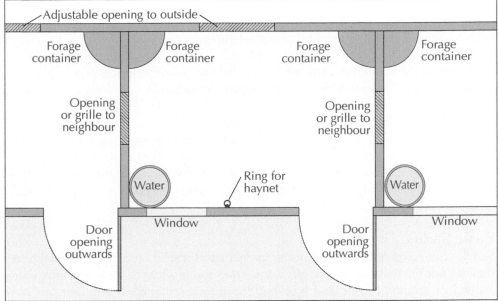

82 A suggested layout for horse friendly, environmentally-enriched stabling. The horses stabled in this set-up will be able to see out from front and back and at least sniff and touch noses with their neighbours through the grilles in the walls. Friendly horses can be stabled in large stables together or at least with a separating partition that is just above wither height. There is a selection of different fibrous feeds or forages for them (at least three types). This mimics, to a small extent, the variety they have when grazing and enables them to wander from source to source according to what they want, as they do when free. There is ample water and, although not shown here, the feed and water containers are fixed low down so that the horses eat and drink naturally with their heads down, which makes for comfortable eating, contentment, drainage of airways and effective digestion.

I am greatly in favour of providing feed containers in all corners of the stable filled with different sorts of forage (fibrous) feed so that the horses have plenty of variety, partly mimicking their natural grazing facility.

In cases where horses genuinely need to have more restrained access to friendly neighbours, grilled chat holes at least should be present in the dividing walls so the horses can see and sniff each other and touch nostrils.

TACK

The sense of touch is clearly involved when a horse wears tack and other equipment. The one *sine qua non* to be observed in this whole milieu is that the horse must be comfortable if he is to work well and to rest and relax adequately in his off-duty time. Horses are not able to concentrate fully on what they are being asked to do if they are troubled by discomfort or pain anywhere in their bodies or if they are anxious in their minds. Similarly, clothing (see Clothing) is worn for many hours at a time and can cause horses significant distress if unsuitable. The nerve endings/receptors affected by contact with equipment are those for touch, pressure and pain.

Whatever aiding system is used, the object of all good riding is that the horse should be schooled ultimately to respond to the lightest possible touch of rein and leg, including contact with the bit. The seat applies pressure through the saddle, if one is worn. Pain can be experienced by a horse if the rider uses harsh methods or if the tack is adjusted too tightly or in other ways incorrectly.

A general guideline for tack and equipment for ground work, riding or driving is that you should be able easily to slide a finger under all straps all around. You should be able to slide the flat of your four fingers under girths, surcingles and rollers without being able to pull them far away from the horse's side, and under and around saddles when the horse is not mounted.

Basic Saddle Fit

Saddles can cause significant and sustained discomfort and, in certain cases, actual pain if they do not fit. This can be a result of squeezing and pinching, uneven pressure, sliding around or creating friction and bruising. Pressure concentrated in one area can cause swelling and bruising and, over time, if not corrected, atrophy (wasting) or even necrosis (death) of the affected tissues due to restriction of the local blood supply. This sort of event can occur because of poor fit, uneven stuffing or padding, wrong sizing, inappropriate design for the horse concerned, or carelessness such as folded under panels and numnahs, wrinkled pads and dirt and debris rubbing into the horse. Also, the discomfort or pain can easily cause defensive behaviour during work, which can prove dangerous.

Saddles should be fitted and regularly checked by a qualified saddle fitter. When the horse's heaviest rider is in the saddle, you should be able to see a clear channel of daylight down the gullet from pommel to cantle and fit the width of three fingers underneath the front and rear arches. Any more and the saddle may be perching due to being too narrow; any less and it may be sitting too low due to being too wide. In the first case it will pinch and cause excessive pressure, and in the latter it may rock around and cause bruising.

A common fault with many saddles today is that they have very flat panels under the seat and 'bridge' on the horse's back, pressing more in front and behind and less in the middle. When the rider is in the saddle, his or her weight presses the saddle down on the horse's back and the uneven pressure becomes even worse. A saddle should always follow the smooth curving line of a horse's back. Most horses do not have flat backs.

Another fault is that many people set their saddles too far forward. The saddle should be placed so that the front edge of the front arch (the pommel) is behind the top of the shoulder blade, just behind the withers, to the extent that you can fit the edge of your hand between the two (83–85). At the back, the saddle should not extend past the horse's last rib onto the loins. If the saddle is positioned comfortably and is well designed and fitted, it will sit on the horse's back so that the lowest part of the seat is in its centre and the rider can sit there, not be constantly drawn towards the cantle with the legs thrown forward.

This positioning should also help to ensure that the girth is not pulled too far forward into the horse's elbows, digging in there with every movement of the forelegs. Restriction of the shoulder blades and elbows is very uncomfortable for the horse and will ruin his willingness to move freely forward. Extra padding is not the answer; it will make a tight saddle even tighter and is just a stop-gap for an overwide one.

Rather than buying girth sleeves (which will not stop the pressure under the elbows), it is preferable to buy a couple of girths that are cut away behind the elbows, making sure the cutaways are in the right places by measuring the horse before ordering the girths. Girths that have elastic inserts at both ends or in the middle are more comfortable for the horse and they create an even rather than a lopsided stretch when the horse breathes in.

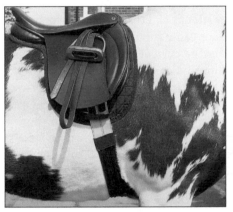

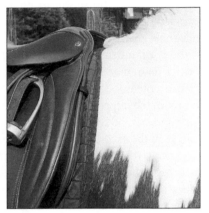

83 A good quality, well fitting saddle for general riding (suitable for flatwork and negotiating moderate jumps). It is placed far enough back from the tops of the shoulder blades (just below the back of the withers) to allow free shoulder movement in action and also free foreleg movement, because the girth is lying a little way back from the elbow. The saddle is of such a length that it does not press on the horse's loins at the back.

84 This saddle, in itself, fits well at the front and allows space for the standard three fingers' width between the pommel and the horse's withers, but the numnah beneath it is right down on the withers. This will cause considerable pressure on this sensitive area when a rider's weight is in the saddle.

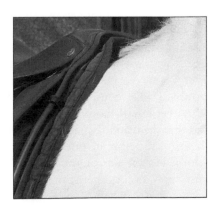

85 The same saddle with the numnah pulled well up into the saddle gullet all the way along. In this way it will not cause pressure on the withers when the horse is ridden.

Fit of Bridle, Bit and Noseband

As mentioned above, you should be able to slide a finger easily under all the straps of the bridle. You need to be able to fit the width of your hand between the throat latch and your horse's round jawbone (restriction here discourages the horse from 'giving' to the bit). The headpiece must be narrow enough to sit comfortably behind the horse's ears without rubbing them. Therefore, the browband must be long enough to allow this, but not so long that it flops about and irritates the horse. The cheekpieces of the bridle and noseband must be well away from the horse's eyes and not rub the horse's facial bones.

Whatever type of noseband is used, remember that you must be able to slide a finger easily all around the horse's head under the straps, including over the nasal bone, and the straps must not restrict the horse's breathing, as horses are able to breathe only through their nostrils. The noseband must not cause rubbing or pressure on the horse's facial bones or, indeed, anywhere else (86). The current fashion in some quarters for tight, often extremely tight, nosebands cannot be conducive to a horse's comfort nor does it promote good horsemanship. It actually causes distress to many horses, as can be seen from the expression on their faces (87), sometimes their difficulty in breathing, and the tendency of some to grind their teeth (a sign of distress) and to show general discomfort in the area constricted. My personal opinion is that using nosebands (or any tack) in such a restrictive way is a welfare issue. As far as quality, skilled horsemanship is concerned, this way of using nosebands prevents a horse correctly and gently mouthing the bit or relaxing and flexing his jaw at the temporomandibular joints just below the ear, so 'giving' his lower jaw to the bit.

Fitting Bits

The following points may be helpful in achieving comfort and, therefore, a more cooperative attitude and improved equine welfare and performance. Although the position of the horse's teeth should be considered, basically:
- Jointed bits should normally make only one wrinkle at the corners of the horse's mouth (86–88).
- Straight-bar or half-moon/mullen mouthed bits used alone (i.e. not as part of a double bridle) should comfortably touch the corners of the mouth without making any wrinkles, but not be so low that the horse shakes them about or gets his tongue over the mouthpiece. The curb chain or strap, if a pelham or Kimblewick bit is used, should lie flat and right down in the curb/chin groove, not ride up above it. You should be able comfortably to slide one finger along under it, and it should come into effect when the lower cheek of the bit is brought back to an angle of 45 degrees with the line of the horse's lips. If looser than this, it has little effect and, therefore, encourages the rider to pull on it.
- A double bridle, consisting of a bridoon or bradoon (thin snaffle) and a curb bit with either a half-moon or ported mouthpiece (with a shallow hump in it) should fit so that the bridoon makes one wrinkle and the mouthpiece of the curb lies about half an inch below it, not touching the corners of the mouth. In the mouth, the bridoon lies on top of the curb mouthpiece. The same remarks about the curb chain apply as for a pelham.

86 The correct height for a jointed snaffle bit, in this case a loose ring type. The bit is creating just one wrinkle at the corners of the mare's lips. The noseband is a simple cavesson style, which is loose enough to allow a finger to be slid under it all around the jaws. Note that this mare's muzzle vibrissae or whiskers have, correctly, been left on. She is quite comfortable with her bit, her muzzle being relaxed and soft.

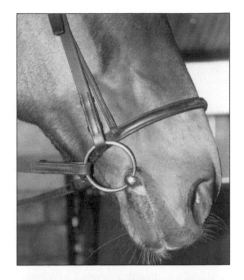

87 The same horse as in 86, but the mare's unhappy facial expression says everything. The bit has been adjusted too high, a common practice that causes horses a lot of discomfort and even pain. Her nostrils are wrinkled up and back, she is grinding her teeth, she is tense and she is trying to get her tongue over the bit to avoid the discomfort. Her eyes also show her anxiety.

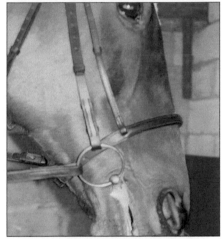

88 The correct height for a non-jointed bit, fitting snugly up to the corners of the lips, but creating no wrinkles. The curb chain is lying correctly down in the curb or chin groove and comfortably touching the skin. It is adjusted so that it just comes into effect when the bit's lower cheek is drawn back to an angle of 45 degrees. This is a Rugby Pelham bit without the headstall on the bridoon ring. Again, note that the muzzle is quite relaxed because the mare is quite comfortable with this, her normal bitting arrangement.

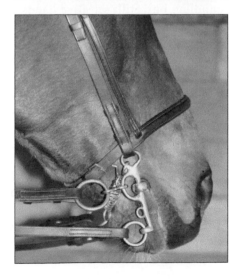

• As for width, you should be able to fit the width of one finger between the horse's cheek and the upper cheekpiece or ring of the bit on one side, so that the bit neither pinches nor slides around.

It is often found that horses who have become hard or dull in the mouth (not usually their fault, but that of poor, insensitive riding) respond better to a change of bit that lies in a different position, acts differently and makes the horse think. Some horses respond to a constant change or to different bits for different pursuits.

Bitless Bridles

There are various designs of bitless bridle available, from simple side-pull bridles to strong leverage bridles with long cheeks. Some act almost entirely by means of pressure on the nose and some act on the whole head. While many horses go well in them, and they can be very handy to use in cases of a bit injury, not all do so. Sometimes, a constant change from one design to another, creating different sensations, keeps a horse's responses 'fresh', as with changes of bit.

Some horses seem to benefit from being ridden in a bitless bridle and a conventional bridle, alternately. Again, this seems to introduce an element of refreshing change and keeps the horse mentally on his toes. Much depends on the mentality and attitude of the horse, which are partly integral to him and partly a result of his previous experiences, good or bad. Some horses do just seem to want to 'get away' with not cooperating and they perceive a bitless bridle as the rider having little or no control. Other horses are quite amenable to bitless bridles. They work better without the risk of being hurt by a bit or the sheer uncomfortable feel of a bit in the mouth. (It is as hard to say that horses do not mind having bits in their mouths as it is to say that humans do not mind having to wear dentures. Horses clearly look relieved when their bridles and bits are removed. They often mouth and lick noticeably, as well as rubbing their heads on humans or haynets and looking for food and water.)

Leverage bitless bridles, which work by pressure on the nasal bone and the poll, can be very strong in their action and are by no means a substitute for lack of skill in handling bits. Still, sensitive hands are needed to operate them effectively and safely without causing the horse pain and even injury.

Good Horsemanship and Applying the Aids

The tack a horse wears can be quite comfortable if care is taken over its fit and adjustment, as described above. The purpose of the tack is to give the rider a more comfortable and secure seat than he or she could have riding bareback, and it is a means of better control of the horse via the bit and reins. Some types of horsemanship do not rely on bits. Many primitive peoples used variations of ropes and hide strips around their horses' heads, with a single rope to the hands. Rawhide or ropes were then passed through the mouth and two reins were thought of and, finally, bits (of wood, bone, horn and metal) were invented for even more control.

Many people ride today without bits or anything at all on their horses' heads. There is nothing new about this and it says a great deal for the relationship riders have with their horse and their ability to use mainly their seat and legs to aid the horse (89–91).

89 A good leg aid. The leg is down with the toe forward, which maintains a stable position in the saddle. The aid is given with the whole of the inside of the leg (not just the heel) pressing sideways against the pony's side in an on-off movement.

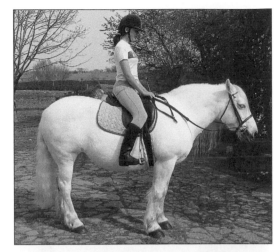

90 A bad leg aid, and very common. The rider has raised her thigh and turned her toe out, which takes the inside of the leg away from the saddle and destabilizes her seat. She has put her leg back from the knee (rather than using the whole leg) and is pressing into the pony's side with the back of her heel. This has bad effects on the rider's finesse and stability.

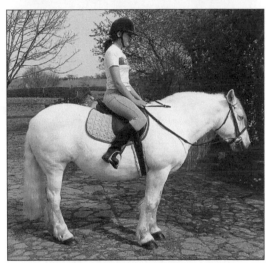

91 A good leg position seen from behind. The leg is dropped and draped lightly against the horse's side without significant pressure, ready to be used or not, as required. Constant heavy pressure with the legs against the sides, or aids given at every stride, dull a horse's responses.

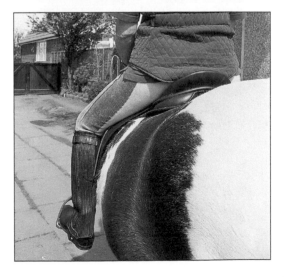

There are many levels and standards in training horses, from completely green (beginner horses) to very advanced ones. The traditional aim of quality equitation is to have a horse moving at least as well under saddle as he does without a rider and, eventually, to enhance his natural way of going (92–97).

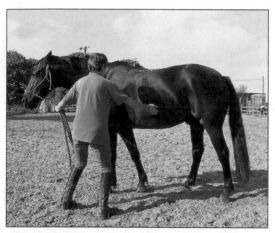

92 Training a horse from the ground to respond to pressure on his side. To move the horse's hindquarters over and away from the handler, press or tap lightly on his side and say 'over'. The horse has moved his right hindleg over and is about to follow up with his left hindleg. From the saddle, putting the leg back from the hip, applying the aid and giving the command (the horse now being familiar with both touch and sound) will (or should!) result in the horse moving his hindquarters over.

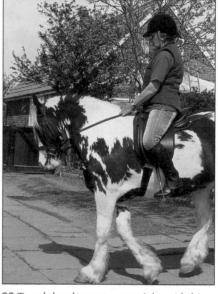

93 To ask her horse to turn right with his weight on his hindquarters, the rider has put some weight onto her right (inside) seat bone and down her right leg into her stirrup. She has put her left (outside) leg back to stop the horse's hindquarters swinging left and is pressing sideways with her left rein on his neck just in front of the withers. There is no pulling on the inside rein. The horse turns easily.

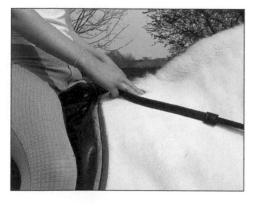

94 A subtle and easy way to ask your horse to turn is to push or tap with the fingers of your outside hand against his withers. Horses quickly come to understand this aid and turn willingly.

95 The inside aids for a good turn are to weight your inside seat bone and stirrup a little, give the outside aids (see 93) and invite the horse round with an open rein aid with your inside rein. This rider's wrist is turned so that the thumb is pointing outwards. This old, classical aid seems to enhance the light, turning effect of the inside rein. The whole picture is much more attractive than pulling the horse round in an unbalanced way with the inside rein.

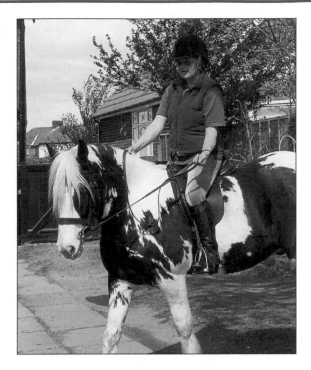

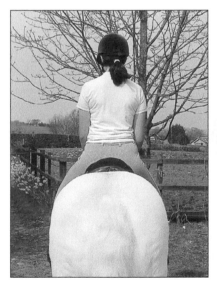

96 This rider is sitting square (balanced and level) on her pony's back, the saddle, too, being placed centrally on the pony. This position allows for even, effective weight distribution and application of weight aids.

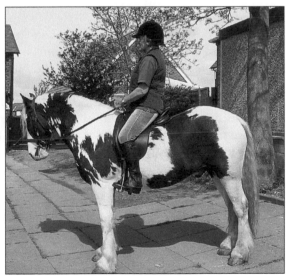

97 A good, balanced classical seat. You could draw a straight line from the rider's ear, through her elbows and hips and on down the back of her heels. She is sitting balanced on her seat bones and, if you pulled the horse away from under her, she would land on her feet, not her bottom, a traditional criterion of a correct position.

Also, depending on his rider's interests, the horse may be required to perform various movements such as jumping obstacles, racing around barrels or performing simple or more intricate patterns on the ground with his body held in such a posture that it will be strengthened to enable him to carry weight (his rider) with little effort and to move in self-balance or self-carriage. All this, done effectively, can take years of training, depending on your aims, but it produces a light, balanced, usually cooperative horse who is a joy to ride and who gives every appearance of enjoying his work.

With conventional tacking arrangements there are several aiding systems, both formal and informal. The whole point, for humane and effective riding, is to get your result without causing the horse pain or discomfort. Applying any aid involves applying pressure with the hand on the mouth, head or neck, with the legs as pressure against the horse's side, or via weight from the seat on the horse's back, either directly, if bareback, or through the saddle.

As with any pressure, unremitting or rapidly repeated pressure reduces or 'wears out' the sensory nervous response, a process also known as adaptation. The production of the chemical neurotransmitter that diffuses across the synapse between two nerve endings 'runs out' and needs a little restoration time for optimal sensitivity and function to be renewed. However, several mechanisms account for the weakening of the 'message' transmitted from sense organs to the CNS, exhaustion of the neurotransmitter being only one. The timescale for recovery (as well as exhaustion) may be too quick to account for the waning of the horse's response to the leg aids. In any case, the horse will certainly feel something on each kick, even if some classes of skin receptor have adapted.

When a rider constantly presses or rubs his or her legs against the horse's sides, kicks him with or without spurs and thinks he or she has to be 'doing something' at every stride to keep the horse going, the horse's sensitivity dulls, as it does when constant, firm and even hard mouth contact is maintained. In this case the reason involves a behavioural change (learning) afforded by the neuronal plasticity of the brain. In time, you can end up with a hard-mouthed, dead-sided horse who is no pleasure to anyone to ride. Just as importantly, the horse can surely have no interest or pleasure in this situation, which is not his fault. Mentally, he must regard the constant nagging and interference from his rider as par for the course, and because it does not 'say' anything specific to him, being constantly present, he ignores it.

There is a better way. Applying an aid only when you want the horse to perform or start a particular movement, and gradually during training applying it lighter and lighter so that the horse ultimately responds to a whisper of an aid, will create the willingness and lightness sought by every empathetic and skilled horseman and horsewoman. For example, with leg aids, once you have your result, stop the aid, sit there and enjoy it. Do not think that you have to keep applying it to make the horse keep doing it. If the horse back pedals or stops executing your request (e.g. drops into a walk when you have asked him to trot), then reapply the aid, possibly with a vocal command as well, but stop it as soon as the horse trots and say 'good boy'. The consistent and instant release of the aid tells the horse that the pressure will stop when he trots. Ultimately, this forms a habit and the horse complies with a light aid almost without thinking.

This is only one example, but it does set out the general idea of establishing a light aiding system. If there is no cessation of pressure, however light, the horse gets no relief from it by having done what he perceives as necessary to stop it (trotting on). Also, if, like me, you believe that horses do understand when you are pleased or displeased with them, if you do keep asking despite the horse having performed what you asked for, he cannot know (a) that he has done the right thing or (b) that you are pleased. This must be mentally confusing and frustrating and even, in some horses, a cause of anxiety. Ask for the trot with a light inward squeeze of your legs just behind the girth (a very sensitive area) that lasts no more than a second. Do not put your heel up and back and keep it pressed or grinding into your horse's side till he obeys; that does not make for lightness. Repeat the quick squeeze with a vocal command and maybe a simultaneous light tap with your schooling whip behind your leg until the horse trots. Then stop it immediately and praise him instantly so that he connects the cessation of pressure and the praise with the action. This method retains the nervous function, confirms to the horse that he was right to trot and lets him know that you are pleased. By riding with your body in trot mode you maintain the trot; you do not have to keep telling the horse to do it.

The rein and bit aids work similarly. Unfortunately, many people are taught today to keep up a very firm contact with the horse's very sensitive mouth, which will soon become very insensitive with this treatment. As mentioned earlier, the nerve endings could be destroyed by traumatic overstimulation. This would be physical damage, in contrast to sensory adaptation or even learning. It is hard to say that most 'hard mouths' are due to such damage, though it is possible that the more usual mechanism is the unlearning of responses to rein and bit aids. Many riders also concentrate on having the horse's neck shortened up and in, and the front of his face on or behind a vertical line dropped to the ground from his forehead. This firmly held position, combined with the hard bit contact (not to mention the tight noseband described earlier), results in the horse's head and neck being held in a vice-like grip, all of which is exactly contrary to high-quality horsemanship as laid down in the best texts on good riding and taught by the best teachers.

There is a better way to do this, as well. In riding, the outside rein (the one on the outside of any bend or circle you are executing) is your master rein. It controls the speed and guides (but should not force) the horse's posture. The inside rein asks the horse to flex (bend or look) in a particular direction and also to 'soften' or flex his jaw and accept the bit lightly in his mouth. An old and proven rule is not to use both reins in the same way, as this feels constricting to the horse and can cause many to resist, putting you on the first steps along the road to a hard mouth and a heavy ride.

The outside rein (or whichever rein you choose if on a straight line, such as riding down a road or track out hacking) should be held with the same amount of pressure (contact) as you would use to hold the hand of a small child whom you are taking across a road; firm enough for control but gentle enough to be comfortable and reassuring. This pressure should not be absolutely constant and unrelenting, but be like elastic, variable according to the circumstances. (The minutiae of riding techniques according to circumstances are outside the remit of this book.) The inside rein should be held with a slightly lighter contact, ever ready to transmit little vibrations or squeezes to communicate to your horse what you want him to do.

With rein contact, keep it 'there' with the outside rein, gently firm and supportive, and give gentle but definite squeezes on the mouth via the inside rein to ask the horse to flex at the poll and 'give' with his lower jaw (which inevitably means opening his mouth slightly). When performed by a reasonably sensitive rider, this will result in a horse working well, with his neck stretched out forwards and, maybe, arched upwards as well if more advanced, dropped or flexed comfortably from the poll so that the front of his face is somewhat in front of the vertical line described above, and with his lower jaw comfortably relaxed and opened slightly from the temporomandibular joint. This enables him to work and accept his bit comfortably.

With positive and tactful brief squeezes from the rider's legs (particularly the inside one), and voice and manner, the horse will learn to flex his lumbosacral joint to bring his pelvis and hindlegs more under his body and to slightly increase the natural arch of his spine. All this can be done with willingness and give the horse enjoyment in his own paces, without the distress and discomfort engendered by the demanding, forceful riding often seen today. There is no constant, unrelenting pressure on the horse's mouth or sides, so he remains lightly responsive to the aids and learns to go in self-balance under a still, balanced rider from fairly early on in his education, making further progress quicker and easier.

Using your weight to create pressure on the horse's back is also an aid that horses understand instantly. Where you put your weight (and often where you look), your horse will go. To 'tune in' to this kind of classical riding, simply be aware of your seat bones and sit on them, not back on your buttocks. Let your legs drop down, using your stirrups to support them on the balls of your feet, and position your ankle bones immediately beneath your seat bones on a vertical line viewed from the side. To enhance your balance even more, imagine this line starting at your ear, running down through your shoulder, elbow and hip and through your ankle. Concentrate your awareness between your hips and accept that your seat bones are where the control comes from.

As you are walking your horse on a straight line, just move your right seat bone forward in the saddle slightly. Also, put a little more weight on your right seat bone and down your right leg, pressing lightly into your right stirrup, with the weight dropping down and out through your heel. Do not tilt your upper body; rather give yourself the feel of stretching your right leg downwards. Your horse will move right, needing no other physical aid, but more so if you look there as well. Release the pressure and he will straighten up. Try it again to the left.

Once your horse is used to weight aids, you can simply move your seat bones where you want him to go. You will get superb results with this natural aid, which horses are quite happy to obey provided you do not stop them by some other means such as pulling on your outside rein or pushing sideways with your inside leg. You can also teach a horse 'right' and 'left', by saying the words as he is moving in whichever direction.

HANDLING

The sense of touch in handling can make the difference between calm, cooperative success or abject and possibly dangerous failure. Always remember to be calm, firm and positive, and this should apply when in the saddle and when on the ground. When you touch a horse, it should instil confidence in him, calm him down, encourage him, liven him up or let him know that you are in charge of the situation.

Stroking a horse on the lower neck and withers area calms him down, causes a drop in heart rate and is therefore excellent for diffusing potentially fraught situations. This is particularly so if you can persuade the horse to lower his head so that his poll is lower than his withers. When horses are excited, worried, angry or frightened, a firm stroke coupled with lowering the head and, if possible, finding something to distract the horse from whatever is occupying and frazzling his mind and concentration (e.g. getting him to look or go elsewhere), are proven successful ways of restoring order.

It is always better to stroke horses rather than pat them in such situations. Stroking is similar to mutual grooming. A firm stroke with the hand or a rub with the knuckles on the lower neck and withers feels like the scraping and nuzzling another horse would give when grooming. On the other hand, patting feels like the short, sharp, unpleasant feel of a horse nipping or biting as a natural, aggressive gesture to get another horse out of his space. Therefore, it is inappropriate for delighted riders to thump and slap their horses hard when they have done well.

There is still much talk about horses being 'into pressure' animals (sometimes incorrectly termed 'inter pressure'), meaning that they lean into pressure. This has significant implications, for example, for horses pulling against a consistent bit contact (which they do) or leaning on an aid (from the saddle or the ground) that does not let up. Horse do lean into steady pressure of this sort, but they definitely back off from intermittent pressure.

When a horse appears to be crowding you, either intentionally or otherwise, a good way to move him away from you, if he will not respond to a light touch on his side or whichever part of him is too close for comfort, plus the word 'over', is to jab him with the end of your thumb supported on the side of your index finger and your hand formed into a firm fist. Often, one jab with the thumb will send a thoughtless horse away a little, but you may need to do it a bit harder and repeatedly for a horse who is not responding. This is an effective and harmless way of protecting your own space and is similar to what horses do to each other with their teeth, so it is readily understood.

Using a similar technique (intermittent pressure) usually works well when trying to gain more cooperation from horses who are slightly difficult in hand, who will not walk on when required or who halt or back (98, 99). Give gentle or firmer quick tugs on the headcollar or halter lead rope (about two per second), so that the horse feels repeated, intermittent pressure on his poll, and keep it up till he realises that the only way he can relieve himself of the pressure is to move his head away from it, either by placing his head down or moving forwards.

To get the horse to halt in hand, tug as described above backwards on the lead rope so that he feels the intermittent pressure on his nose. This also works if you want the horse to go backwards, as does a hand patting firmly on his chest or, in more difficult situations, the end of your thumb jabbing on the bone low down on his chest.

The key point to remember for success is that you must stop the pressure the instant the horse does what you want, otherwise he cannot learn that he has done the right thing. If you want him to move further in whatever direction you are asking him to, and he has stopped, wait a couple of seconds and then repeat the process.

What about using vocal commands as well, and praising the horse? Once the horse has developed the habit of obeying the aid in various places, so that you know he is responding to the aid and not merely associating it with a particular place such as his stable, as he is moving as required give an appropriate vocal command such as 'walk on' or 'back' so that he associates that sound with that movement. Pretty soon, you will only need to say what you want and the horse will develop the habit of doing it without a physical aid. To get to this point you must be absolutely consistent with this training so that the horse always knows where he stands and can rely on consistency from you. It is useless to do it on one occasion but not the next.

When the horse is responding as you wish, all you have to do, as you stop your aid, is say in a very pleased tone something like 'good boy', 'there' or whatever you choose, but be consistent with this, too. Consistency and a calm, firm, positive attitude are crucial to any kind of horse handling or training.

CLOTHING

Horse clothing can be a curse or a blessing. A good range of clothing can be a real help in keeping a horse comfortable year round, but there does not seem to be a good understanding of how it should fit and how much harm can be done to the horse's mind and body when it doesn't. The size of the rug or blanket is only one aspect that should be considered. If the design and shape do not suit the body type of the horse for whom it is intended, it can cause too much pressure and friction and, therefore, discomfort and even distress to that horse. One angle on clothing that is also often overlooked is that horses wear it for many hours at a time, so the discomfort and discontent that can be caused can be long lasting.

98 A nose chain can be used with animals that are difficult to lead in hand. They must be used only in an intermittent pressure way (i.e. on-off) and not be a sustained feel. They must also not be used to tie up a horse. This photo shows the lead rope clipped to the rings of the chain, not the headcollar, for correct and effective use.

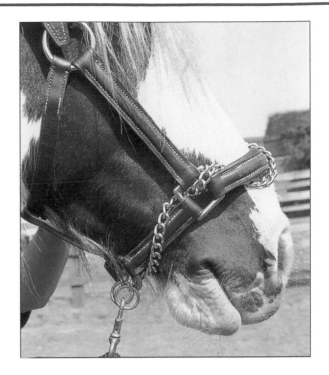

99 The nose chain from the front, showing how it is wound around the noseband of the headcollar. It is passed through the side dees and then through the jaw ring.

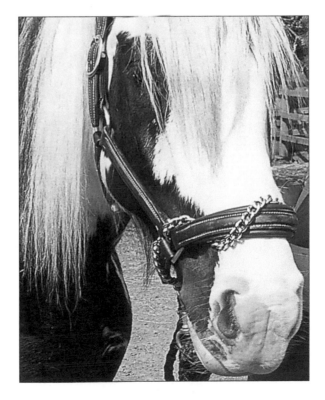

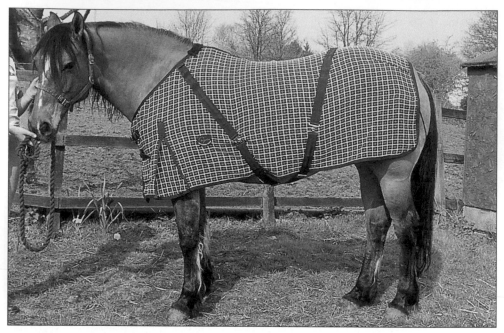

100 This rug is quite well fitting. It comes well in front of the withers and has inserts at the elbow to allow room for movement. There is no need for it to be any deeper, as it is a summer weight rug, and it comes well back over the hindquarters, with a fillet string behind the thighs to help to keep the back part in place.

Today, most rugs/blankets are cut in the shape of the horse's body, with an undulating back seam and pleats or darts at the hip and shoulder to allow for not only shape but also movement. Many rugs, both cool weather and cold weather ones, are of the duvet type and although they do not need a spine-shaped back seam, they do need to make room for the horse's withers, shoulders, croup and hips, and for his movement (100). This applies whether they are indoor rugs for stable use or outdoor ones for use in a paddock or field.

The most common areas in which rugs cause friction and pressure are on and around the withers, the points of the shoulders, the croup and the hip bones (wings of the pelvis). When you look at a rug on a horse, look for areas where the rug is clearly pinched for room; for example, where it is clearly pulling tight (usually on the areas mentioned), has radiating folds running from a pressure point, is so tight that you have difficulty in running the flat of your hand inside it between rug and horse, or is digging into the horse's neck and, therefore, pulling down hard on his withers when he tries to get his head down to graze or root in his bedding. These are all signs of a badly fitting rug or blanket.

Depending on the country concerned, rugs may be sold in imperial or metric gradations of size. To measure your horse for his size, use a tape measure or a piece of string. Place one end in the middle of the horse's chest and run the tape around his shoulder and along his side to the back of his thigh where his tail hangs. This gives you the size. When purchasing, tell the seller the type of horse you have (e.g. Thoroughbred, cob, native pony, finer show pony, warmblood, heavy horse) and say that you are concerned about the design type as well as the size. Some of the duvet-type rugs will fit almost any horse if the size is right, but make sure that they have really generous pleats or 'cut-outs' on the bottom edge around the shoulder and stifle area to ensure that the horse can move around, lie down to rest or roll, get up and, if out, gallop around without his action being interfered with. Some horses who feel uncomfortable in their rugs are discouraged from moving around and from lying down to rest, which is clearly contrary to their welfare and general health.

When the rug is in place, the neckline needs to come up around the base of the neck and lie in front of the withers, allowing plenty of room to run your hand and arm freely between the rug and the shoulders. At the back the rug should come to the root of the tail, although outdoor rugs need to come a little past it. The bottom edge needs to be down to the elbows, maybe longer in an outdoor rug. Finally, make sure that the breast fastenings allow the horse to get his head down in comfort without undue pressure on his neck and withers, that any belly strap is snug but neither tight nor loose, and that the leg straps, if present, permit you to fit the width of your hand between them and the horse. Linking them through each other, after making sure they are not twisted, helps to ensure that they feel comfortable in this area of very sensitive skin.

Signs of badly fitting rugs and blankets, apart from their appearance, are ruffled disturbed hair, bald patches, changed behaviour in the horse, disturbed and rubbed mane around the withers and a horse who starts biting at his clothing or stands looking uncomfortable, although the latter can also be a sign of illness (e.g. colic or laminitis).

Rugs should be changed at least twice daily for ones of different design in order to provide a change of feel and pressure for the horse. Some pressure is unavoidable. The point is to make sure that the pressure is reasonable and does not cause any of the symptoms described above.

ELECTRIC FENCING

Electric fences stimulate a variety of nerves directly. The sensations felt are likely to be due to the signals sent to the brain as a result of these nerves firing in response to the electric field, although stimulation of the nerve endings or receptors may also play a part.

Horses are adept at foiling electric fencing. Some may charge through the fence and some 'crawl' under the fence; some need 'high-dose' electricity to deter them; some chew the insulators on top of removable posts; and a number learn that when there is no audible tick the fence is off and they are virtually free.

One point about electric fencing, which is difficult to overcome, is that if a horse grazing near it flicks his tail and catches the wire, he will get an electric shock. This is fine if he skips away from it, but if the tail wraps around the wire, tape or one of the posts, he can become caught up and career, panic-stricken, around the paddock pulling the fencing with him. This may be a rare occurrence, but it has happened, and makes a good case for the more permanent type of firmly fixed fencing rather than the temporary sort, however useful and mobile the latter may be.

White electrified tape is used a great deal and is easy for horses to see. Other types of electric fencing can be made safer by tying strips of coloured or white plastic to the wire to warn horses of their presence.

To introduce horses to electric fencing, the common method is to moisten their muzzles, lead them up to the wire and surreptitiously and lightly touch the muzzle against the wire. Repeat this in a couple of places and the horse will soon be reluctant to go near the wire. However, this procedure may result in the horse creating a bad association with the handler/owner, and it may be preferable to simply let the horse discover the electric fence by himself.

PROPRIOCEPTION

Proprioception is the ability of a horse (or any animal) to sense his own body position and movements from information transmitted by sensory nerve endings that respond to stimuli within the horse's own body rather than outside it. It is enabled by the horse's nervous system, but it is also closely allied to the balancing organ of the inner ear. The proprioceptive sensory receptors are sited in the labyrinth of canals in the inner ear, in the joint capsules of the skeleton, and in tendons and the skeletal muscles that move the bones of the skeleton.

This ability is crucial if the horse is to be able to move effectively, and the horse uses proprioception all the time. The special nerve endings are stimulated when the horse moves in any way; for example, when he stretches, when he is deciding where to place his head, limbs or body for his own purposes or when asked by a handler or rider, when he wakes up and wants to get up, when jumping to avoid hitting a fence, when travelling so that he can keep his balance, or when he wants to lie down and roll.

A horse, like other animals, finds it easier to keep his balance if he can lean on or even just touch a fairly still, stable support. When his body moves or is moved by the motion of a vehicle in which he is travelling, he can use the support of the side of the vehicle, the partition, a firm breast or breeching bar or even the breeching strap to help him sense how and in what way his body has moved or been moved. This tells the horse how to position himself in order to remain on his feet. Horses, as prey animals, are very loath to fall down. Many horses lean in this way during transport. Many driving horses use their vehicle as a means of support to help them to balance. This is possible because the vehicle is separate from the horse and 'connected' to the ground (to some extent, at least, depending on the amount of friction between wheels and ground). Driving horses may lean on the pole, the shafts or their partner in a pair.

In the case of ridden horses, the rider is part of the same inertial frame as the horse. There is no outside contact other than that of the horse's feet with the ground, so there is no outside force upon which to lean. This would be like us wearing a backpack with two straps that we hold. We could pull against the straps, but we could not use them to stop us falling over because the backpack moves with us. It is not possible, therefore, for a rider to 'hold up' or 'support' a horse via the bit, and the consequences of trying to do so can be unpleasant for both horse and rider and counterproductive to good riding and schooling.

The support that some riders and trainers believe they are giving to a young horse by means of firm bit contact is not support, as such, at all. Horses, both young and mature, ridden in this way become 'heavy in hand', being ultimately somewhat insensitive to the bit. They also do not learn to 'carry' themselves, but are constantly working against the restriction of the bit. This is why, in good riding, horses are taught from early on to develop their own balance. In much modern riding, as described earlier, the rider wants, and is taught, to be the horse's prop by means of an overfirm bit contact and an apparently purposely restricted head and neck. The rider shows a real reluctance (I find as a teacher) to let go and gradually allow the horse to learn to balance himself under his weight and to start learning to go from a lighter contact. This is possible even in horses with already hard mouths, as the horse uses other sensory means to decipher from the rider's aids what he would like him to do.

The reason horses have problems balancing themselves under some (probably most) riders is that the rider is not sitting and moving in balance with the horse. Horses can balance themselves perfectly well when free, and if they have problems when mounted, it can only be because of the rider; nothing else has changed. This is a big subject outside the scope of this book, but it is a crucial one. It is why the traditional system of the best riders riding and schooling the young, green horses and the made horses 'teaching' the novice riders is definitely the best.

The rider, too, relies on proprioception to keep himself balanced after he has sensed what the horse is doing with his body. The only supports the rider has, his feet not being in contact with the ground, are the feel of the horse's trunk through his seat and legs and of his head and neck through the bit. The rider can sense the horse's movements and can move his body appropriately not only to keep his balance on the horse's back but to influence the horse as to what to do with his body, where to go and how.

The subject of proprioception has been dealt with very fully by TDM Roberts (1995). Like other abilities, balance and proprioception work on a 'use it or lose it' basis. The more you use these sensory nervous abilities the more highly developed they seem to become. It is surely best for both horse and rider to be self-aware physically and able to balance independently. The horse needs to learn self-balance under weight and it is the rider's responsibility to keep that weight as stable and helpful to the horse as possible. Only when the rider can adapt his or her movements to those of the horse in such a way as to not interfere with his natural movement is he/she in a position to influence him by means of the aids. Most horses and riders come across situations such as riding over rough ground, in tricky places, trying to 'see a stride' to a jump and riding in poor light conditions. In such situations the ability of both of you to use proprioception and independent balance to keep yourselves upright and safe could be crucial to avoiding a fall.

THERAPIES

There are several therapies involving the horse's sense of touch, but I have chosen just three to describe because these particular ones are appropriate for owners to apply themselves with a little study and common sense.

Hand Rubbing

Hand rubbing is a traditional practice that was carried out in good stables until a couple of generations ago; however, it may have gone out of fashion due to time constraints in the modern world. Few people now know about this practice and as it is so simple and good for the horse, relaxing him, stimulating his skin and superficial muscles, perhaps drying him off and encouraging circulation, it would be well worth reviving (**101**).

It is a very simple practice in which the groom (this term encompasses anyone caring for the horse) simply uses his or her hands and forearms to rub the horse down after work or gently during illness, injury or convalescence; it can also be performed as a pre-work stimulant. It depends on whether you do it briskly and firmly or more slowly and lightly. Obviously, injured areas should be avoided.

Wearing a short-sleeved top, or rolled up sleeves, stand with your feet a little apart to give yourself a firm base of support and, using both hands and forearms, start at the shoulder and rub the horse confidently and sensitively all over. If there are any areas about which he is touchy, go carefully, leaving them and perhaps coming back to them later when he may well be enjoying his rub down so much he will let you treat him there.

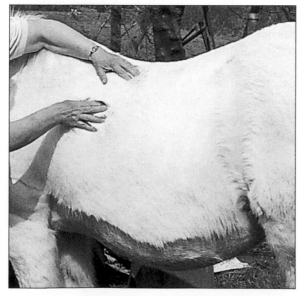

101 Hand rubbing is an old and comforting way to give a horse a light massage, to dry him off if damp and to treat his muscles after work.

If you are giving a stimulating or after-work toning rub down, put your weight behind your hands and arms by leaning on to them, and work briskly. If you are dealing with a sick or injured horse, do not use much weight and work more slowly. Let your hands mould to the shape of the horse's muscles and body and be careful over bony areas. Concentrate on muscle mass areas, but also cup your hands round his legs and rub them upwards towards the heart. There is an argument for rubbing anywhere on the horse towards the heart to help move on lymph and other body fluids (102), but some horses do not like having their coat hair rubbed 'against the grain'. Many horses also like their faces being stroked and rubbed gently and their ears being 'stripped' (pulled gently from base to tip), which can be very comforting to a tired horse. Also, many horses particularly like being rubbed in areas they cannot reach themselves.

Spend about five minutes on each side, or a little more if you have time and the horse is enjoying it. To finish, stroke the horse all over in the direction of the hair from ears to tail and lightly down the legs.

Massage

Massage is a specialized, professional therapy and a thorough massage from a qualified sports massage therapist or physiotherapist really gives a horse the feel-good factor. There is no reason, however, why owners cannot perform a simplified form of massage; it is really just an extension of hand rubbing. Work on the muscle mass areas and avoid bony areas, the abdomen and the throat.

102 'Chopping' with the sides of the hands on muscular areas of the horse loosens up the tissues and encourages the blood, lymph and energy to flow through them.

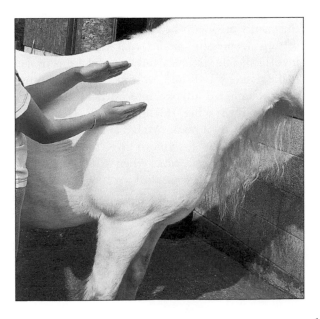

A technique called effleurage is good for an all-purpose massage. It can be used to stimulate or relax according to how you work (i.e. briskly or more gently). You simply place your hands flat but relaxed on your horse and work in the direction of the hair, back and down apart from the legs, which are done in an upward direction to help any fluid that may have collected there to move upwards and onwards. It is normally recommended that you start away from the heart and work towards it, but this means that working from the tail forwards involves rubbing against the hair. Check your horse's response as you work and finish with an all-over stroke to smooth the hair down again.

To apply effleurage, lean the weight on your hands fairly firmly as you push them along the area you are working on, then lift up slightly and bring them back, keeping in touch, but with a lighter contact. Repeat three or four strokes in one place.

Another technique, which is definitely stimulating and loosens up muscles and other tissues, is percussion or tapotement, which you do by making loose fists and bouncing them alternately on the sides of your hands on muscled areas.

You can also use clapping, in which you form little roof shapes out of your hands and clap them alternately up and down, again on muscle mass areas, so that only your fingertips and the heels of your hands actually touch the horse. This makes a characteristic puffing sound with each blow and, as well as stimulating the circulation, it can help to dry off a damp horse.

Shiatsu

Shiatsu is a therapy I recommend a lot. I am a trained equine shiatsu therapist and am fully aware of its benefits as a means not only of health maintenance but also of therapy for physical, psychological and emotional problems. It is a very wide subject, but the basics can be learned by any concerned and sensible horse owner.

Shiatsu is related to acupuncture and acupressure, both of which are now recognized equine therapies and known to be effective. Shiatsu is not massage. It works by means of fingertip pressure (and also, sometimes, the pressure of elbows and forearms) along the energy meridians believed in eastern medicine to be present in all creatures, and on certain acupressure points that can be worked by pressure on them. Shiatsu also involves gentle stretches and manipulations of the body, which can help to loosen and make tissues supple and, to some extent, help correct faulty action.

I recommend anyone interested in shiatsu to buy the book by the late Pamela Hannay (my teacher) (Hannay, 2002). Details of shiatsu and other modalities are also given in my own book (McBane, 2005). But for starters, here is a very basic, general shiatsu treatment for you to give your horse.

Ideally, choose a time when your horse is normally relaxed and not expecting anything such as food, work or turnout. Make sure the stable environment is quiet (i.e. no radios, people laughing, chattering or banging things about, mobile phones ringing). Remove the hay so that the horse will concentrate on the treatment (provided he has finished eating and will not be concerned by this). If the horse is wearing rugs, just remove them while you give him an all-over stroke to alert the meridians, then cover the hind part of his body with them before you begin work. As you work back and forth, move the rugs to the forehand and back again, to keep him warm if the weather is chilly.

103 In shiatsu, one hand (here the left) is used as the control (or Mother) hand and the other, using the fingertips at right angles to the horse's body, is used to press along the meridians. Here, the bladder meridian is being worked.

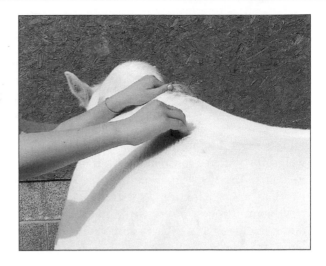

The meridians are believed to be the routes along which flows the body's energy or life force, called 'qi' (pronounced 'kee'). They are mostly named after organs in the body and they enhance the function of the relevant organ. Because a major benefit to general health and healing is to rid the body as far as possible of toxins, a basic shiatsu session will probably involve the stimulation of the bladder and kidney meridians. Note that the bladder meridian runs from front to back and the kidney meridian runs from back to front of the horse. Therefore, the format of a basic and general, owner-applied treatment using meridians would be:

1. Stroke the horse all over with alternate hands, always keeping one on the horse to keep the energy connection. This opens up the meridians in preparation for the next stage.
2. For meridian work you have one hand as your control (Mother) hand, which keeps contact with the horse, and the other as your working hand. To work the bladder meridian, stand on your horse's left side and, placing your left, control hand over the top of his neck (easily resting there), use the palm of your right hand to follow the line of the bladder meridian. Just press lightly on it for a second, then move on, press again, move on, and so on. Your control hand can move to the withers as you work further back, then perhaps the hip, so that you are comfortable but staying in contact with at least one hand.
3. Keeping a hand on your horse, go round to the right side and repeat.
4. Come back to the left side, place your control hand and then follow the meridian, using not the palm this time but the very tips of your fingers held in a line (103), lightly but confidently, and with healing intent, pressing down into where you feel the meridian to be. Stay open and let the feel of the energy come to you. I work intuitively, but some shiatsu practitioners say that they can actually feel the energy flowing under their fingers. Repeat on the right side.

5. Next palm and work the kidney meridian with your fingers in just the same way, all the time thinking about healing and staying quiet, relaxed and confident.
6. To finish, stroke your horse all over again to close down the meridians. As a sign to a horse that I have finished, I pick up the dock and gently pull my hands all the way down the hair, and let it drop. Horses I treat regularly then know that this is the end of the treatment. I do this when hand rubbing or massaging as well.

Horses unused to bodywork may wander around and not concentrate, but they may well settle within a few minutes. In time they will relax and stand free. If a horse new to shiatsu therapy starts walking around after having been still, this is a sign that he has had enough for now, so stroke him and stop. When a horse has had a full treatment, it is best not to work him for 24 hours, the length of time believed to be taken for the energy cycle to complete itself. However, he can certainly be led out in hand or turned out.

Touching in any therapy, provided it is done with healing intent, affection and concern for the horse, is enormously beneficial and therapeutic. Therapists other than those interested in eastern arts are now working partly on the basis of energy flow, and my experience tells me that shiatsu and related techniques are definitely comforting and effective complementary therapies.

CONCLUSION

I hope you have enjoyed reading this book and that it has given you food for thought in relation to how our horses perceive the world we all live in and, maybe, given you a new perspective on caring for and working with horses.

Research continues and I believe that it is our responsibility to keep up to date and to keep on learning as much as we can about horses and our interactions with them. Attitudes change and although horses undoubtedly do work very hard in many cases, and do not always seem to be managed or ridden appropriately for the kind of animal they are, there is also a noticeable increase in the number of people wishing to find different and better ways of co-existing with them.

Understanding how their bodies and minds function can only give us an enlightening view of the inner world of horses and how they cope with their external world, often perceiving it very differently from how we do. We can help them a great deal by being more understanding and by caring for, training and working them in better ways than we often do now.

Please let this book take you on to more knowledge about these amazing creatures, some of the largest and most sensitive on our planet, who probably only still exist because they are so useful and attractive to us.

FURTHER READING

Currently there are many excellent horse books being published. The following list indicates those books that the author feels will be found thought provoking by readers attracted to this book. Some of the books in the list are not new publications, but there is a very great deal to be learnt from them if trouble is taken to seek them out, perhaps from libraries, second-hand bookshops and antiquarian dealers. Many book retailers operate a book search for out-of-print books and the internet is a source of all books, old and new.

Budiansky S (1997) *The Nature of Horses: Their Evolution, Intelligence and Behaviour*. The Free Press (a division of Simon & Schuster, USA) and Weidenfeld & Nicholson (an imprint of The Orion Publishing Group), London.

Davies Z (2005) *Introduction to Horse Biology*. Blackwell Publishing, Oxford. (Also, any other books by this author.)

Downer J (1988) *Supersense: Perception in the Animal World*. BBC Books (a division of BBC Enterprises), London.

Fraser AF (1992) *The Behaviour of The Horse*. CAB International, Oxford and New York.

Gray P (2002) *Essential Care of the Ridden Horse (The Indispensable Guide to Achieving Optimum Health for your Horse)*. David & Charles, Newton Abbot. (Also any other books by this author.)

Hannay P (2002) *Shiatsu Therapy For Horses*. JA Allen (an imprint of Robert Hale), London.

Heuschmann G (2007) *Tug of War: Classical versus 'Modern' Dressage – Why Classical Training Works and How Incorrect 'Modern' Riding Negatively Affects Horses' Health*. JA Allen (an imprint of Robert Hale), London.

Kiley-Worthington M (2005) *Horse Watch: What It Is To Be Equine*. JA Allen (an imprint of Robert Hale), London. (Also any other books by this author.)

Loch S (2000) *Dressage in Lightness: Speaking The Horse's Language*. JA Allen (an imprint of Robert Hale), London. (Also any other books by this author.)

Macuda TJ and Timney B (2000) Wavelength discrimination in horses. *Investigative Ophthalmology & Visual Science* (Supplement), 41:S809.

McBane S (1999) *How Your Horse Works*. David & Charles, Newton Abbot.

McBane S, Davis C (2001) *Complementary Therapies for Horse and Rider*. David & Charles, Newton Abbot.

McBane S (2004) *100 Ways To Improve Your Riding: Common Faults and How to Cure Them*. David & Charles, Newton Abbot.

McBane S (2005) *Bodywork For Horses*. Sportsman's Press (an imprint of Quiller Publishing), Shrewsbury.

McGreevy, Paul and McLean, Andrew, *Equitation Science*, (Wiley-Blackwell, 2010), ISBN 978-1-4051-8905-7

McGreevy P (2004) *Equine Behavior: A Guide for Veterinarians and Equine Scientists*. WB Saunders (a division of Elsevier), Philadelphia. (Also any other books by this author.)

Mills D, Nankervis K (1999) *Equine Behaviour: Principles and Practice*. Blackwell Science, Oxford.

Rees L (1984) *The Horse's Mind*. Stanley Paul, London.

Roberts TDM (2006) *Recollections of a Frustrated Scientist*. Published privately and available from the author for £15 sterling including postage and packing. (Contact Dr TDM Roberts at 11 Holmehill Court, Smithy Loan, Dunblane, Scotland, FK15 OAF.)

Roberts TDM (1992) *Equestrian Technique*. JA Allen (an imprint of Robert Hale), London.

Roberts TDM (1995) *Understanding Balance: The Mechanics of Posture and Locomotion*. Chapman and Hall, Andover.

Skipper L (2003) *Realize Your Horse's True Potential*. JA Allen (an imprint of Robert Hale), London. (Also any other books by this author.)

Thorn PF (1949) *Humane Horse-Training*. Hutchinson, London.

Waring GH (2003) *Horse Behavior* (2nd edn). Noyes Publications/William Andrew Publishing, Norwich, USA.

Williams M (1990 and later editions) *Understanding Nervousness in Horse and Rider*. JA Allen (an imprint of Robert Hale), London. (Also any other books by this author.)

Wright M (1973) *The Jeffery Method of Horse Handling*. Published privately by Maurice Wright, Dyamberin, Armidale, Australia.

Zeitler-Feicht MH (2004) *Horse Behaviour Explained: Origins, Treatment and Prevention of Problems*. Manson Publishing, London. In USA, Trafalgar Square Publishing, North Pomfret VT.

INDEX

T - #0447 - 071024 - C160 - 234/156/7 - PB - 9780367381776 - Gloss Lamination